KEY QUESTIONS IN HEALTHCARE LAW AND ETHICS

Sara Miller McCune founded SAGE Publishing in 1965 to support the dissemination of usable knowledge and educate a global community. SAGE publishes more than 1000 journals and over 800 new books each year, spanning a wide range of subject areas. Our growing selection of library products includes archives, data, case studies and video. SAGE remains majority owned by our founder and after her lifetime will become owned by a charitable trust that secures the company's continued independence.

Los Angeles | London | New Delhi | Singapore | Washington DC | Melbourne

KEY QUESTIONS IN HEALTHCARE LAW AND ETHICS

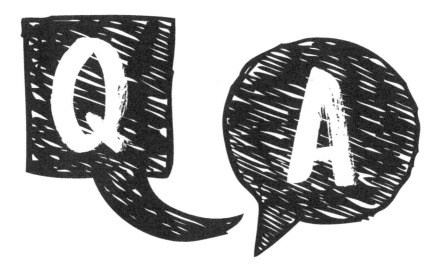

MARC CORNOCK

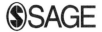SAGE

Los Angeles | London | New Delhi
Singapore | Washington DC | Melbourne

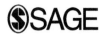

Los Angeles | London | New Delhi
Singapore | Washington DC | Melbourne

SAGE Publications Ltd
1 Oliver's Yard
55 City Road
London EC1Y 1SP

SAGE Publications Inc.
2455 Teller Road
Thousand Oaks, California 91320

SAGE Publications India Pvt Ltd
B 1/I 1 Mohan Cooperative Industrial Area
Mathura Road
New Delhi 110 044

SAGE Publications Asia-Pacific Pte Ltd
3 Church Street
#10-04 Samsung Hub
Singapore 049483

Editor: Alex Clabburn
Assistant editor: Ozlem Merakli
Production editor: Tanya Szwarnowska
Copyeditor: Salia Nessa
Proofreader: Jill Birch
Marketing manager: George Kimble
Cover design: Wendy Scott
Typeset by: C&M Digitals (P) Ltd, Chennai, India
Printed in the UK

Library of Congress Control Number: 2020946110

British Library Cataloguing in Publication data

A catalogue record for this book is available from the British Library

ISBN 978-1-5264-6343-2
ISBN 978-1-5264-6344-9 (pbk)

At SAGE we take sustainability seriously. Most of our products are printed in the UK using responsibly sourced papers and boards. When we print overseas we ensure sustainable papers are used as measured by the PREPS grading system. We undertake an annual audit to monitor our sustainability.

To Nan and Dad, this is for you.

And also for Mum, Simon and Siân.

Scarlett Neville, I am sorry that I distracted you on Christmas Day. You should know by now that if you ask me a question, I will probably give a lecture as an answer. This book is my apology; I hope it is useful to you in your studies.

CONTENTS

DETAILED TABLE OF CONTENTS

LIST OF TABLES

LIST OF CASE NOTES

ABOUT THE AUTHOR

Marc Cornock is an academic lawyer and Senior Lecturer in Health in the Faculty of Wellbeing, Education and Language Studies, The Open University. Before this, Marc was Senior Lecturer in The Open University Law School, and prior to that was Principal Lecturer and Academic Lead for law in health care in The Faculty of Health and Social Work at the University of Plymouth.

During a professional career within healthcare, Marc undertook a master's degree in medical law and a PhD at Cardiff University Law School, and studied undergraduate law at The Open University.

Marc's teaching interests lie in both general law and in health law. Marc has lectured on legal aspects of healthcare to various professional groups. His research focuses on the interface between the law and healthcare practice, and he has written extensively on this for professional and academic audiences.

AUTHOR'S ACKNOWLEDGEMENTS

I would like to take this opportunity to formally say thank you to the many people who have assisted me in the development of this book from its initial conception, through development and writing, to its actual production.

Many students and colleagues have allowed me to develop my thinking on health law and I am thankful to all of them. In particular, the year 3 nursing students on the BSc (Hons) Nursing programme at the University of the West of England who attended the 'extra AMC' classes and those who participated in the health law seminars at the University of Plymouth.

My thanks to my colleagues at the University of Plymouth for their support in developing health law and ethics into distinct areas of teaching within the curriculum. I am keen to single out Dr Andrew Nichols, lecturer extraordinaire at the University of Plymouth, for his invaluable contribution to the development of this book. Andy has spent considerable time and effort in assisting me with the development of a book based on questions we were asked in lectures, seminars and talks that we gave on law and ethics to healthcare students during our joint teaching sessions. I am eternally grateful to him for all his time, and the talks and discussion we have had over the years regarding law and ethics in general and in relation to this book.

I would also like to express my sincere thanks to Andy for permission to use his notes for the basis of Chapter 5.

To my family and friends, thanks for putting up with me during the writing phase of this book: even if you didn't know that was the reason I wasn't available or was not always in the best of humour.

Finally, but never last, Sarah. Words will never be able to express my gratitude for everything you did and do, so I have gone with the simplest and fewest words (as my unofficial editor, that's what you always said you wanted in my writing!), thank you.

Marc Cornock
West Yorkshire
November 2020

PUBLISHER'S ACKNOWLEDGEMENTS

The publisher is grateful to the following academics for their work on reviewing the proposal and draft material of this text:

Peter Ellis, Independent Nursing Educational Consultant and Writer

Thomas Walvin, University of Plymouth

INTRODUCTION

This book is a bit different to many you will pick up. So, I have written this introduction to explain what it is about and the approach I have taken when writing it.

This book grew out of my teaching sessions with various groups of healthcare practitioners on health law and ethics. In my teaching, it became apparent that different groups of healthcare practitioners shared the same anxieties and dilemmas regarding their practice; such that similar questions were emerging in all the teaching sessions.

This book answers those common questions.

Now a word about what the book is *not*. It is not a formal textbook on health law and ethics; it is not a dry list of questions with equally dry answers. I have endeavoured to make the answers as simple and interesting as possible so that you can get to the root of the problem quickly; and it is not a comprehensive review of health law and ethics, rather it covers the common questions that I have been asked, the ones that you may want to ask, the ones that everyone assumes that everyone else knows.

It has been written so that it will be appropriate for all levels of healthcare practitioner – from the learner, in the initial stages of their education, to the advanced practitioner who wishes to refresh their knowledge, or maybe learn something new.

What is unique about this book? It is based around a question and answer approach. If we were able to sit down and chat, this is what you may ask and how I would answer. The approach taken in each of the chapters is to avoid large chunks of indigestible material by using questions that ensure all the important information is covered. Each chapter is structured but in a way that allows you to easily find what you may be looking for. There is no need for you to start at page 1 and read to the end, though feel free to do so if you want. You can go straight to the question you want answered and read that. Most of the answers are short(ish) although one or two are notably longer because of their complexity.

SOME 'HEALTH WARNINGS'

Throughout the book, the word 'patient' has been used as shorthand for clients, patients and individuals in receipt of care and treatment from healthcare practitioners. Similarly, 'healthcare practitioner' is used as shorthand for anyone who provides care, treatment, advice, counselling, guidance or in other ways meets the health and care needs of patients. It is used for all grades of practitioner and all professional groups. Where a law or guidance or policy refers to a specific practitioner group, for example paramedic, this word will be used.

(Continued)

There is no separate chapter on the child, and legal and ethical issues relating to the child. This is because the students I have worked with prefer to have issues relating to the child taught at the same time as that relating to adults. Therefore, information relating to the child is in the same chapter as that for adults.

There is no index to this book. The list of questions in the **detailed table of contents** will hopefully assist you in finding the information you are looking for, as the questions are written in a manner that indicates what is addressed in the answer as well as being written in the language that they were asked.

Oh, the bold bit in the paragraph above. I need to explain that to you. Sometimes to answer a question I need to refer you to another question. To do that I will put the question you need to refer to in bold. Of course, it's up to you if you do but it's my suggestion of where you may find additional information.

The structure of each chapter follows a familiar format. There is an introduction to what the chapter will discuss; a list of questions that will be addressed; the questions and answers; a summary of the main points and a reference list. Where the details of a legal case may help to understand a specific principle, the details will be presented in a box separate to the rest of the answer.

You can think of this book as having three parts. Part 1, which is actually Chapter 1, is the foundation for all that follows; it provides an introduction to ethics and the law, the relationship between the two, and considers how they both affect the practice of healthcare practitioners as a group and as individual healthcare practitioners. For those unfamiliar with ethical and legal principles and the sources of law in the United Kingdom, it provides the essential background information which will clarify the issues explored in the remainder of the book.

Part 2, Chapters 2 and 3, builds on the fundamentals of law and ethics to outline the environment in which a healthcare practitioner works and the standards, rules and regulations which both constrain and permit their practice. While each chapter in Part 3 (the remaining chapters), is a comprehensive account of an aspect of healthcare ethics and law, for instance consent or confidentiality, that healthcare practitioners may face in their practice and decision making.

A QUICK WORD ON LAW AND ETHICS

Chapter 1 is, as you may guess from its title, an introduction to the subjects of ethics and law. If you are happy with them as subjects, feel free to skip Chapter 1. If on the other hand, you are not so sure or you want a refresher, Chapter 1 is for you.

What I want to point out is that after Chapter 1, law, ethics and indeed regulation is mixed in the questions that follow, except where it is explicitly referred to separately. By 'mixed' I mean that I don't refer to an ethical aspect and a legal aspect of a specific issue. This is because in healthcare practice they are integrated and overlap, and this is the approach I have adopted. What you will find in this book is that, because of the sanctions that can occur, the practical application of law has a stronger focus and will come through in the book.

In this book I have adopted an informal chatty style of writing so that the information should feel related to the actual work that you do. In your practice I am sure, because I have seen your colleagues do it and been told by my students that they do it, that you have a laugh, a joke and are informal with your patients when the situation allows for it. Doing so alleviates many patients' fears and stresses. This is how I undertake my practice too, only my practice is teaching. I try to have an informal atmosphere in my teaching rooms and allow my students to direct as much of my lectures as I can. The style I have used in this book is an extension of this; I think that my students learn best when they are relaxed with the subject. The answers I provide in this book are the answers I would provide to you if you asked the question in my lectures, seminars and workshops. In fact, they contain more information than there is usually time to cover!

However, don't be fooled into thinking that the informal approach is superficial in its covering of subjects, or I am not serious about the subject or its consequences. It is possible to be both serious about a subject but also to be informal, and at times irreverent, about it. The informal approach and use of questions allows each subject to be divided into manageable chunks, which are not dry and distant from the work you do. You could read through a chapter using the questions as your guide, or if you are looking for the answer to a specific problem, use the list of questions to determine where the answer will be found.

I hope that you find this book to be informative and interesting, but also enjoyable. I welcome any comments you may have. I would be keen to hear if there is a question that you would have liked to have asked, or something extra you would wish to be included in an answer. Let the publisher know, I am sure they will tell me.

Thanks for reading this far.
Marc

AN INTRODUCTION TO ETHICS AND LAW

Chapter 1 introduces ethics and the law, the relationship between the two, and considers how they both affect the practice of healthcare practitioners as a group and as individuals. For those unfamiliar with ethical and legal principles and the sources of law in the United Kingdom, it provides the essential background information that will underpin the issues explored in the remainder of the book.

Throughout the chapter/book, the term 'state' is used to mean a country that is able to govern itself and so issue its own laws and decide upon its own regulatory mechanisms.

QUESTIONS COVERED IN CHAPTER 1

- Why are ethics and law important?
- What are ethics?
- What is the law?
- What are the traditional ethical theories for healthcare?
- Are there any limitations of the traditional ethical theories?
- How have healthcare ethics been reconsidered?
- What are the main ethical principles relevant to healthcare practice?
- Where does law come from?
- What is the role of the Courts?
- What is the difference between criminal and civil law?
- Why is the law so confusing?
- How do ethics and law affect me?

 Q Why are ethics and law important?

A Ethics and law are important aspects of healthcare practice because they provide the foundation upon which practice can develop.

Healthcare is a unique profession because of the relationship between the health-care practitioner and the patient. Although patients are involved in their own healthcare needs and care, there can be an imbalance between the two parties. In any such situation, there needs to be a framework or guidance as to how the person with the perceived power, the healthcare practitioner, should act in relation to the other person, the patient, and what is and is not acceptable behaviour. This is the role that ethics and law play, through the development of principles, in healthcare delivery. Ethics and law apply to healthcare practitioners, their practice and their relationships with patients.

As well as setting the framework within which healthcare practitioners must undertake their practice, it forms a key element of this book: how ethics and law support the healthcare practitioner to undertake that practice.

Ethics and law are not a single entity, although they may be said to be inter-twined in most spheres, such as in healthcare, where the one supports the other. In order to understand the relationship between the two concepts, we will firstly explore the two separately and then consider how they relate to each other.

What are ethics?

A dictionary definition of ethics is 'the science of morals'; 'the rules of conduct recognized in … human life' and 'the science of human duty in its widest extent' (Onions, 1984).

Although morals and ethics are related in that one can inform the other, they are distinct from each other. Morals may be seen as a standard of behaviour whereas ethics are more of a system for understanding this behaviour.

Morals relate to the individual, being based on the individual's religious, societal or personal beliefs; how the individual views their actions in a given situation; and whether they see something as being good or bad. For instance, one person's morals may mean that they believe telling a lie is always wrong; whereas another person's morals mean that they see lying in some circumstances as justified, what is some-times known as the 'white lie' concept.

Ethics are based on morals in that they can affect and control the actions of individuals; however, they are a formalised system of accepted or acceptable beliefs about how individuals within a particular group should act in a given situation. Ethics allow for personal beliefs to be shared within a given group and to be system-atically developed for the benefit of the group.

There are several ethical theories that provide guidance for a person's actions and behaviours; two of these are discussed in **What are the traditional ethical theories for healthcare? (p. 6)**.

What is the law?

Although 'the law' is a very common expression, what do we mean when we talk of the law?

The law is a system of rules. Rules that govern the operation of society, for instance what government can and cannot do, as well as governing the individuals within that society through the development of accepted behaviour. There are various forms of rule that exist in any given society.

Etiquette is a form of rule that governs how individuals act toward each other, yet if someone was to breach the rules of etiquette it is unlikely that they would find themselves subject to the might of the legal system. Custom can also be seen as a set of rules; rules that are recognised by particular groups of individuals and govern their behaviour, for instance religions have customs that affect how their followers practise the religion. Other rules apply to the society as a whole rather than a subset within that society. They are the rules that society expects all individuals within the society to observe. Laws are an aspect of society's rules. However, whereas the non-observance of a custom or rule of etiquette may result in a sanction by members of the subset of society who follows them, the non-observance of a law results in a formal sanction by society against the individual.

The fact that certain rules are elevated to the status of laws means that society holds them in higher regard. As such, these laws are enforceable through the legal system, which includes the police service and the Courts. The purpose of the legal system is to ensure that the rules are followed and that anyone who does not follow the rules is dealt with appropriately. Whether this is through the criminal or civil legal system, the outcome is that the 'wrongdoer' faces a sanction that is imposed through the legal system, the Courts. It is said that, as well as being a punishment for the 'wrongdoer', the sanction should act as a deterrent to others who are considering breaking the rules of society.

Law is state specific. It is related to the particular characteristics of the state and also to a point in time. As the society evolves, so do the laws of that society, so that the law represents the contemporary society's view of acceptable behaviour. However, one feature of the law of the United Kingdom is that laws do not go out of date; unless they are specifically enacted for a limited period of time only, laws remain in force until they are repealed. Thus, in the United Kingdom today, there are laws that have been in existence for hundreds of years, sitting alongside the laws that are enacted in each passing year.

Law allows society to function. At the simplest level, law governs the relationship between the individual and the state. In return for certain rights, for instance the right to vote, society demands certain obligations from the individual, for instance not committing a crime (or as a lawyer would say, a criminal offence – why use one word when you can use two!).

What are the traditional ethical theories for healthcare?

There were two ethical theories that were traditionally taught and considered to be relevant to healthcare practitioners and to healthcare itself. These are Deontology and Utilitarianism. Here we will look at both of these theories in the way that they were presented, that is as a binary approach to ethics: something was approached through either a deontological or utilitarian outlook.

DEONTOLOGY

Deontology literally means the study of duty. It arises from the Greek for duty, 'deon'. As an ethical theory, it can be traced back to the work of Immanuel Kant, a Prussian philosopher working in the mid to late 1700s. Kant's philosophical theory is grounded in what he termed the 'categorical imperative'.

A categorical imperative is something that has an intrinsic nature about it that is good. No external validation is needed to make them good. For humans to be morally good, they have to follow all categorical imperatives. Therefore, a categorical imperative becomes a selfless act; it is something that has to be done because of a duty or obligation to do so. Duty or obligation are key underlying features of deontology as Kant believed that if someone acts without there being a duty to do so, there is no moral value to that action.

One aspect of the categorical imperative is that individuals should always act as if their action was to become a universal ethical law for others to follow; that is to act without any personal motive.

Someone who acted according to deontological ethics would do so because they felt they had a duty or obligation to do so. They would have no free will in the choice of action but would feel compelled to act in a certain way. Thus, actions can be classified as being good or bad according to the reasons behind the act. Failing to act when there is a duty to do so would be seen as behaving unethically.

Therefore, for deontologists, clear duties and obligations exist in given situations. For instance, the healthcare practitioner who is off-duty but comes across someone who requires their assistance would have a clear duty to act for the benefit of the individual rather than themselves (see **Do I have a duty to individuals outside my clinical practice? [p. 44]**).

In this way, codes of practice can be said to have a deontological ethical basis, as they require the individual subject to them to act in certain ways because of their duty or obligations. Indeed, the Health and Care Professions Council's (HCPC) *Standards of conduct, performance and ethics* (Health and Care Professions Council, 2016) actually begins with the words 'Your duties as a registrant' (title page). Each of the ten standards that make up the 'code' then begins with the words 'You must'. The Nursing and Midwifery Council's (NMC) code has a similar approach, with its introduction stating that, 'The code contains the professional standards that registered nurses, midwives and nursing associates must uphold' (Nursing and Midwifery Council, 2018: 2). Similar to the HCPC code, each of the 25 standards in the NMC code start with 'To achieve this you must'. It is only after the duty has been stated do the codes provide any guidance as to how you, the healthcare practitioner, who has to use and follow them, may achieve the duty.

When considering how to act in any situation, the person acting according to a deontological ethical perspective would ask, 'What is my clear duty in this situation?'. Not, 'What *should* I do?', or 'What do I *want* to do?' but 'What do I *have* to do?'

UTILITARIANISM

Utilitarianism developed through the late 1700s and the early 1800s, and was generally influenced by two British philosophers, Jeremy Bentham and John Stuart Mill. It is also known as consequentialism (for reasons that will soon become apparent).

Compared with deontology, utilitarianism is said to be a much easier ethical theory to understand. Its basic premise is that an act should be based on the premise of maximising utility and minimising worthlessness: or to put it another way, doing the greatest good and the least harm. Thus, any action is judged, not by it being a universal right or wrong as in deontology, but on the outcome it produces. The consequences of the action are the key aspect of any act in utilitarianism/consequentialism.

Those actions that result in more good than harm are seen as being more ethically desirable in utilitarianism.

Other ways of looking at utility and worthlessness are pleasure or happiness and pain or suffering. Accordingly, utilitarianism is often referred to as 'the greatest happiness principle'.

However, rather than concentrating on pleasure at the level of the individual, the utilitarian theory concentrates upon the greatest happiness for the greatest number of people. If I were to do something that gives me pleasure but causes pain for more people than it provides happiness, this would go against utilitarian ideologies. However, if I can gain pleasure or happiness from doing an act that also gives others more pleasure than pain, this would be in accordance with utilitarian theory.

Therefore, when considering any act, the individual must consider the outcomes in terms of the number of individuals it affects, and the type of effect that it will have upon them, as well as the length and severity of that effect. You should act to cause the greatest good or happiness for the greatest number of people for the longest period of time.

There are two types of utilitarian ethical thinking: the act utilitarian and the rule utilitarian. The act utilitarian considers the nature of an act and the consequences that follow from undertaking the act, or from not undertaking the act, and chooses the decision, doing or not doing the act, that results in the greatest happiness. The rule utilitarian, on the other hand, considers what the outcome would be if the rule, whether to act or not, was always followed. If always following the rule would produce more happiness than always not following the rule, then the rule is followed, and vice versa. The rule utilitarian may be seen to be a cross between the act utilitarian and the deontologist, in that they act for the greatest good but according to a general rule and not on an individually thought out basis.

Are there any limitations of the traditional ethical theories?

Neither of the theories discussed in **What are the traditional ethical theories for healthcare? (p. 6)** provide an all-encompassing ethical theory for every aspect of healthcare practice. Both of the theories have their supporters and their detractors, and both have limitations.

DEONTOLOGICAL LIMITATIONS

Because it is based upon duty and obligation, deontology is seen as being a logic-based principle; it is said to lack the emotional aspect of human thinking and behaviour. In any situation, an individual will not only consider what their duty is as a means of logical thinking, but their emotional intelligence will play a part in their decision making.

Deontology has also been criticised because it does not allow for free will: if, as individuals, we always act according to a duty or obligation, then actions cannot be free as we are just following the universal duty that everyone else is following too.

Another limitation of deontology is that it does not consider the outcome or consequence of an action, just whether there is a duty to act or not.

Thus, for healthcare practitioners, rather than working with and for the individual patient, you are instead just following your duty and doing what is expected of you. Consider all the times that you have stayed beyond the end of your shift because there was too much that still needed doing. This was not a selfless act on your part; no, for deontologists this was your duty. In making the decision to stay or not, you had no real choice; you had to stay and help your colleagues on the next shift because otherwise you would not be fulfilling your duty.

UTILITARIAN LIMITATIONS

A key limitation of utilitarianism is that it is very good at considering the effect of an action on a large scale, the greatest happiness for the greatest number of people, but not on the small scale or for individuals. Indeed, strict adherence to utilitarianism can be said to subjugate the rights of individuals and to achieve happiness for the greatest number at the individual's expense. In essence, if the greatest happiness means that the rights of one individual are ignored or even displaced, the strict utilitarian would say this is an acceptable price to pay.

It can be argued that utilitarianism is difficult for the individual to follow because of the difficulty they face in predicting how their actions will affect others to ensure that it will result in more pleasure than pain for the greater number of those it affects. There is also the notion of what is good and that two individuals may have differing, even opposing, views of what is good and thus will act accordingly but with different outcomes.

Another limitation of utilitarianism is that of intent versus outcome. An individual may carry out an action with the intent of causing happiness to a lot of people, but their action goes awry, and they end up causing a great deal of misery. Is this still an ethically acceptable act? If, as the utilitarian believes, an act is ethical because of the fact that it causes more good than harm, the intent is irrelevant and the outcome is all that matters.

If we return to you staying behind after the end of your shift to assist your colleagues, the utilitarian does not consider your intent, the reason why you stayed behind, just whether by doing so your action results in more good than harm.

From the discussion of their limitations above it can be said that neither deontologists nor utilitarianists consider the person to be important in ethical decision making, as they either consider they have a duty to act a certain way or that it is not their intent in acting but the outcome that is important.

This and the other limitations discussed have resulted in a re-evaluation of ethical theories in healthcare practice.

Q

How have healthcare ethics been reconsidered?

A

As we saw in **What are the traditional ethical theories for healthcare? (p. 6)** and **Are there any limitations of the traditional ethical theories? (p. 9)**, neither of the two traditional ethical theories can provide an all-encompassing framework that would cover all healthcare situations and guide you in your actions and decision making.

To do this they would have to at least be combined but, as their approach is mutually exclusive (deontology does not consider the consequences of undertaking a duty and utilitarianism is based on the consequences of an action), this is not possible. As a way of addressing the limitations and inadequacies of a binary approach to ethical practice and decision making, virtue ethics and rights-based ethics have gained more prominence in recent years.

Virtue ethics, which have their origins with Aristotle, move away from deontology and utilitarianism in that they are concerned not with a duty to act or the outcome of an act, but rather with the reasoning behind why someone acts. Virtue ethics sees individuals as having a sort of moral compass (their virtue) that will lead them to making the right choice in a given situation. For the healthcare practitioner, virtue ethics recognises why they are making a decision, the values and beliefs that the healthcare practitioner has, and their desire to achieve an outcome that is appropriate for the patient.

Whilst virtue ethics does address some of the issues inherent in deontology and utilitarianism, it does raise its own challenges. If virtues and motive are key to deciding on a particular course of action when faced with a dilemma, where an individual lacks the ability to comprehend the dilemma fully, although they may act in a virtuous way, they could act in a way that leads to a wrong outcome. For instance, a healthcare practitioner may not appreciate that others are less virtuous than they are and will lie to achieve what they want. Thus, a patient addicted to painkillers may lie about their condition and/or their level of pain (we will leave aside the debate on whether an addict should be provided with the substance of their addiction or not). If the healthcare practitioner lacks the knowledge or skill to treat someone with an addiction, then even though they may be acting virtuously and for the right reasons, they may unwittingly provide the addict with painkiller drugs that they do not need.

Rights-based ethics are based on the premise that all individuals have certain rights that they can expect to be respected. However, in order for their rights to be respected, an individual has to act in such a way that respects the rights of others. Where there is a right, there is a corresponding duty on the person claiming the right.

Within the healthcare context, we will see in **Why is consent important in health-care practice? (p. 67)** that autonomy (see **What are the main ethical principles relevant to healthcare practitioner practice? [p. 12]**) is fundamental to patient treatment. If the healthcare practitioner wishes to be autonomous themselves, they have to respect autonomy in their patients.

An issue with rights-based ethics is whose rights would be paramount if there is conflict and whether rights are absolute or if they can be subjugated. To go back to autonomy, many healthcare practitioners will have faced the situation where a young child refuses an injection, but the parent wants their child to have the injection. We will discuss the legal situation when we consider **Can a child refuse treatment? (p. 84)**. For now, we just need to recognise that from a rights-based approach only one of the two, parent or child, can have their right recognised as one will have to be subjugated for the other's to be upheld.

Healthcare practitioners have to navigate themselves through ethical mazes throughout their practice. Virtue ethics and rights-based ethics are useful approaches when a healthcare practitioner is faced with a dilemma but, as we have seen, they have their own issues. There is no single 'right' answer to a healthcare dilemma as they are dependent upon the situation and so no single theory can ever give an answer for every situation.

It is tempting to suggest that healthcare should have its own unified ethical theory or framework. Each ethical theory has something to contribute. A unified approach leads to the issue of what is taken from each of the main theories and how we would address any conflicts between the theories.

If the purpose of ethics is to provide a framework for decision making when resolving a dilemma, and if the theories conflict in their method, is there another way of approaching healthcare dilemmas?

Over forty years ago, it was proposed that, instead of looking for an overarching all-encompassing theory, ethical principles can be used to address dilemmas in healthcare. Rather than there being a right decision based on a specific ethical theory or framework, a healthcare practitioner can use ethical principles to guide their decision making. These principles are discussed in **What are the main ethical principles relevant to healthcare practice? (p. 12)**.

What are the main ethical principles relevant to healthcare practice?

Because no single ethical theory is suitable for all healthcare dilemmas (see **How have healthcare ethics been reconsidered? [p. 10]**), Beauchamp and Childress (2013) have proposed the use of ethical principles to assist healthcare practitioners in their ethical decision making and guide their practice. These are: autonomy, beneficence, non-maleficence and justice.

AUTONOMY

Autonomy comes from the Greek for self-law or self-rule. It refers to being able to make decisions for oneself. To be autonomous, the individual has to be able to make decisions that are not coerced or subject to the will of others.

Respecting a person's autonomy is a key principle in both ethical thinking and the law. For a healthcare practitioner, who may be seen as someone in the position of authority with specialised knowledge and skills, to respect a person's autonomy means treating the person as an individual; respecting their ability to make decisions for themselves; providing them with information to allow them to make decisions; obtaining consent before attempting any procedure or treatment; respecting the person's confidentiality; and adopting a professional approach to the person.

The opposite of respecting autonomy is paternalism; thinking that you, as the expert practitioner, know better than the patient. It is likely that you will know more about the art and science of being a healthcare practitioner and about healthcare practice; however, it is highly unlikely that you will know more than the patient about what their best interests are and how it is served. Healthcare practice is a partnership between you, as the practitioner, and the patient. Only then can the patient be autonomous.

Only a competent person (see **What is the legal definition of competence? [p. 69]**) can be truly autonomous. This is because, if someone is unable to make decisions for themselves, they cannot be autonomous. However, it may be possible for a person to have autonomy with regard to certain aspects of their life and to be non-autonomous in others. For instance, to have autonomy over when they receive treatment but not over the type of treatment offered.

BENEFICENCE

Beneficence refers to doing good. For the healthcare practitioner, beneficence is related to promoting the wellbeing of the patient. Doing things that are of a benefit to the patient, undertaking procedures and treatment that serve the patient's best interests.

A problem arises in determining what is in the patient's best interests. The obvious answer is to ask the patient. Yet, what would be the outcome if the healthcare practitioner wants to undertake a procedure that they believe to be in the patient's best interests, but the patient refuses it? Does the concept of the patient's autonomy override the healthcare practitioner's duty to be beneficent? This issue is addressed throughout this book. For now, it is sufficient to say that a healthcare practitioner is not doing good if they override a patient's rights, such as their right to autonomy.

NON-MALEFICENCE

Non-maleficence is related to the concept of '*primum non nocere*', which literally means first do no harm. The concept proposes that, whatever else you do, you should not harm your patient through your actions; therefore, doing nothing may be better than acting inappropriately and thereby causing harm. It is often thought of as being the same or similar to beneficence. However, the two are quite separate principles.

To act in a non-maleficent way, the healthcare practitioner has to ensure that they know the risks associated with the treatments and procedures they perform, when to perform them and when not, so that they do not cause harm to a patient through unnecessary treatment.

The challenge with both non-maleficence and beneficence is in making the judgement between not doing harm and doing good. I am often asked which is more important, to do good or to do no harm. I would argue that, if you don't do good, you have not left the patient worse off than before you didn't do anything; whereas if you fail to do no harm, you have in fact harmed the patient. By failing to do your non-maleficent duty, you cause harm; by failing to do your beneficent duty, the patient does not suffer.

JUSTICE

Justice as an ethical principle is related to fairness. There are different types of justice. One example is distributive justice, which is concerned with the fair distribution of resources; another is rights-based justice, which relates to respecting the rights of individuals.

In the healthcare context, justice can refer to the obligation of treating individuals according to their need rather than any other criteria; to be just in the allocation of resources, including your skill, time and knowledge. It can also be concerned with providing justice to the wider society, in not wasting the resource you have by treating those who are not in need of your skills.

Resource allocation is often cited as an aspect of justice in healthcare. How can a finite amount of resource be allocated fairly amongst all those in need if there is not enough to satisfy demand? This raises questions about whether it would be ethically right to withhold treatment from those with self-inflicted injuries, for instance those who drink, fall down and injure themselves.

It could be argued that to do so would be in the interests of society by protecting a scarce resource; the alternative argument is that justice is served by treating all those who require treatment, regardless of how they came to need that treatment. The question essentially reduces to whether justice should serve individuals or society. In reality, patients in the National Health Service (NHS) are treated according to clinical need.

Q Where does law come from?

A Having spent some time looking at questions on ethics, it is now time to turn our attention to the other aspect of our introduction to ethics and law – the law. It can be said that the ethical principles (see **What are the main ethical principles relevant to healthcare practice? [p. 12]**) form the basis for the law that has evolved to govern healthcare and the practice of healthcare practitioners. For example, as we will see in the **Consent** chapter (**Chapter 4**), the ethical principle of autonomy has been given a legal basis in the law on consent in healthcare.

There are two main types of law within the United Kingdom: these are legislation and common law.

LEGISLATION

Society has given its law-making ability to Parliament and this is exercised in Acts of Parliament, also known as statutes and, collectively with Statutory Instruments, as legislation. For an Act of Parliament to become law, it has to pass through both Houses of Parliament and be given Royal Assent, which is the formality of the monarch's agreement.

Statutory Instruments are a form of legislation that do not go before the Houses of Parliament. Instead, Parliament sets out the scope and range of the legislation in a parent, or enabling, Act and gives the authority to make the legislation to another body; this can be a Minister of State or a specific organisation.

Statutory Instruments may also be used to modify an Act of Parliament without the need for the whole Act to go before Parliament again. Additionally, Statutory Instruments are a way of issuing regulations that are dependent upon recommendations by professional bodies. As time passes and the recommendations change, the Statutory Instruments can be revoked and new ones issued incorporating the new recommendation, without the need to change the original Act of Parliament.

As an example, The Health Professions Order 2001 gave approval for the setting up of the Health Professions Council (now the Health and Care Professions Council [HCPC]) as well as establishing its functions and the scope of its powers. One of its powers is to make Statutory Instruments; similar legislation exists for the other regulatory bodies.

The power to make Statutory Instruments is seen in The Health Professions Council (Registration and Fees) (Amendment) Rules Order of Council 2010. The schedule to this Statutory Instrument states that: 'The Health Professions Council makes the following Rules in exercise of the powers conferred by articles 7(1) and (2) and 41(2) of the Health Professions Order 2001' (The Health Professions Council [Registration and Fees] [Amendment] Rules Order of Council 2010). For interest, this relates to the maintenance of the register and the fees that the HCPC charges its registrants.

Thus, it can be seen that Parliament has devolved power to the HCPC to make its own Rules and Orders (other names for certain types of Statutory Instrument), in connection with its statutory role. In exercising its authority in this regard, the HCPC's Statutory Instruments must be approved by the Privy Council before they can become law and enforceable. This is because, when devolving power to another body to make laws, Parliament still wants to ensure that there is some form of control and accountability, in this case that oversight is provided by the Privy Council.

On a separate note, since 1973, when the United Kingdom signed the Treaty of Rome which permitted its entry into what became the European Union (EU), the laws and regulations passed by the EU have had an effect in British law. At the time of writing, the withdrawal of the United Kingdom from the EU, known as 'Brexit', has begun but untangling European law from domestic legislation will take some time to accomplish.

COMMON LAW

Common law refers to the situation where there is no legislation that regulates a specific area. When this occurs, the Courts cannot turn to the relevant statute and state the law. Instead, they look to previous cases that have established legal principles in the relevant area of law, known as 'precedent', to see what has been decided, or they look at how statutes have been interpreted in particular cases to see if that may have a bearing on the case before them. Therefore, common law may be seen as the use of judgments in previous cases to decide the outcome in a case before the court. A lower court is always bound by a decision of a higher court.

Common law is an important part of the legal tradition and mechanism of law within the United Kingdom; for instance, in England and Wales, murder is a common law offence as there is no statute defining murder.

 What is the role of the Courts?

As we saw in **Where does law come from? (p. 14)**, a key feature of the legal system within the United Kingdom is its reliance on common law and precedent. As such, it is useful to consider the relative positions of the various Courts.

Courts of first instance hear cases in order to make a judgment or ruling based upon the facts of the case and the relevant law. Appellate courts hear cases on appeal. Their function is not to rehear the case but to consider the way in which legal principles have been applied by the lower courts and to issue judgments on whether this was satisfactory or not.

There are special rules, created by statute, on when a case can be appealed, and which court hears the appeal. In general, there is one opportunity to appeal a case based upon the facts of the case, such as when a relevant point has been overlooked in the initial judgment, and further opportunities to appeal where a point of law is at stake; also, the first appeal is a right, and other appeals after this are based upon being given leave to appeal, or permission, by a court.

The United Kingdom has a hierarchical system of court structure, with the highest court being the Supreme Court; judges that sit in this court are known as Justices of the Supreme Court of the United Kingdom. Prior to the establishment of the Supreme Court on 1st October 2009, the House of Lords was the highest court. Decisions from the Supreme Court, and the House of Lords in historic cases, are legally binding on all other Courts. If a court is bound by a higher court, it means that it has to follow the judgment from the higher court.

The Supreme Court hears cases that are considered to have legal importance. Cases cannot just be taken to the Supreme Court; permission has to first be obtained. The cases heard in the Supreme Court include civil cases for all of the United Kingdom and criminal cases, except from Scotland (the final arbitrator for criminal cases in the Scottish legal system is the High Court of Justiciary). It also hears cases related to constitutional matters such as devolution.

In England and Wales, below the Supreme Court lies the Court of Appeal, with judges known as Lord Justices of Appeal. It has both civil and criminal divisions. Its decisions are also binding on the lower courts. Scotland and Northern Ireland both have a hierarchical system of courts with similar functions.

Next, in terms of seniority in England and Wales, are the High Courts. There are three divisions to the High Court which hear civil cases; the Queen's Bench, Family and Chancery divisions. The High Court hears cases that are brought on appeal from lower courts and more serious cases at first instance.

The lower civil courts are also arranged into a hierarchy; however, this is based upon the nature and amount of the claim being brought. Those that involve considerable sums of money are heard in the High Court; whilst those involving less money are heard in the County Courts.

For criminal cases, the hierarchy of the lower courts is that of Crown Court and then Magistrates' Court. Crown Courts usually have a jury and are presided over by a Judge; they hear the more serious criminal cases. Magistrates' Courts, as the name implies, are presided over by a Magistrate and hear the least serious criminal cases.

In addition to the criminal and civil courts, there are also a range of specialist courts. These include industrial and employment tribunals, coroner's courts, and courts of protection such as mental health tribunals.

Q What is the difference between criminal and civil law?

A The legal system of the United Kingdom is divided into two main areas, criminal and civil. The criminal justice system is concerned with the punishment of wrong-doers and is initiated by the state, whereas the civil justice system is concerned with actions brought by one individual or organisation against another.

There are different Courts for the two areas of law and there are also different procedures used in bringing a case to trial and in the court procedure, depending upon whether the case is a civil or criminal one. We will consider the two areas of law in the context of the England and Wales court system.

CRIMINAL JUSTICE SYSTEM

Criminal law relates to the relationship that exists between individuals and the State. Where a rule is deemed to be sufficiently important, the breaking of the rule (or crime) is classified as a criminal offence and is punishable by the State.

Criminal proceedings are known as a 'prosecution' and are initiated by the State. It is the role of the police to investigate crimes, gather evidence and arrest and charge suspects. The Crown Prosecution Service (CPS) is responsible for the con-duct of the case and taking it through the court system. Once the CPS initiates the prosecution, any decision to continue or discontinue rests with them; the police and any victim are unable to demand its continuance or discontinuance, although any requests, and associated reasons, would be considered by the CPS.

The objective of the criminal justice system is to punish offenders and thereby to act as a deterrent to others. The case is adversarial between the prosecution who bring the case and the defendant who defends it.

All cases will begin in a Magistrate's Court and then either remain there, as approx-imately 95 per cent of criminal cases are heard here, or be sent to the Crown Court.

In the Crown Court, the case is heard before a judge and jury. The jury's role is to decide upon the facts of the case, those presented by both the prosecution and defence teams, and to reach a verdict. The role of the judge is to direct the case according to the law. The judge will advise the jury about the law that is relevant in the case and will allow evidence according to the applicable legal rules.

The burden of proving a criminal case is upon the prosecution, the defendant is not required to prove their innocence. The standard of proof, that is the stand-ard against which the case is judged, is 'beyond reasonable doubt'. In effect, this means that the jury or magistrates must be convinced of the defendant's guilt before they can find them guilty; if there is a one per cent chance that the defend-ant is innocent, they must enter a 'not guilty' verdict. The defence legal team's role is to raise reasonable doubt in the mind of the magistrates or jury regarding the defendant's guilt.

The objectives of the court hearing are to decide, on the basis of the facts and the relevant law, whether the defendant is guilty or not and to punish through the sentences the Court can deliver. Sentences can include imprisonment, fines and community-based orders.

CIVIL JUSTICE SYSTEM

Civil law relates to the relationships between those who have a legal personality. In law, an organisation has a legal personality of its own; so, a National Health Service Ambulance Trust will have a legal personality, as will the individuals who work there. Civil law therefore considers wrongs that occur between these 'individuals' that do not involve other members of society.

Civil proceedings are known as an 'action' and are initiated by the person who alleges they have suffered a wrong against them; although, in practice, it is their solicitors who will issue proceedings. Once the case has commenced, either side can request its discontinuance and, subject to the agreement of the other side, the case can be discontinued subject to certain procedures.

The objective of the civil justice system is to award damages (a monetary amount) or other remedy, to the person who has suffered a wrong, not necessarily to punish the wrongdoer. The aim of the damages is to either put the person back in the position they would have been, had the wrong not occurred, or to compensate them for the wrong. Other remedies include an injunction to stop someone from doing something. The case is adversarial between the claimant who brings the case and the defendant who defends it.

In most civil cases, the case will be heard by a judge sitting alone in either the County or High Court, depending upon the monetary value of the case.

The burden of proving the case is upon the claimant, the person bringing the case. The standard of proof, that is the standard against which the case is judged, is the balance of probabilities. In effect, this means which side's case does the judge prefer.

The objectives of the court hearing are to decide, on the basis of the facts and the relevant law, on a dispute between two or more parties and, where appropriate, to award an appropriate remedy.

Q Why is the law so confusing?

A Like healthcare, the law has its own language that can seem confusing to the outsider.

Legal terminology and words and phrases have not always originated from English. The law has been evolving for hundreds of years and French, or a version of it, was the official language of Royalty and their Courts from the time of the Norman Conquest until around the fifteenth century. This means that many terms still in use today have French origins.

At the same time as French was being used, Latin was the official language of the church. This means that contemporary law uses terms that have their origins in French and Latin. Whilst there have been attempts to reduce the number of seemingly archaic terms in use, many still survive.

Contemporary law is not that contemporary, in that it is not rewritten every so many years and brought completely up to date. A law exists in use until it is repealed, meaning that some of the laws in use today have been around for hundreds of years. Even seemingly modern laws are not that modern. The main law on abortion arises from the Abortion Act 1967, over 50 years ago.

Contemporary law is therefore a blend of historical laws still relevant and in use today, as well as those laws that have been created or amended in more recent times. The processes and structure of the law also owes as much to its past as it does to recent developments.

It is important to realise that the law in the four jurisdictions (countries) of the United Kingdom is not the same on any given subject. For instance, Scotland and Northern Ireland have different mental health legislation to England and Wales. In England and Wales, the Mental Health Act 1983 applies in its entirety, whilst in Northern Ireland only Section 147 applies, the rest of the mental health legislation being contained in The Mental Health (Northern Ireland) Order 1986, as amended by The Mental Health (Amendment) (Northern Ireland) Order 2004. In Scotland only Section 146 applies, with the main legislation for mental health issues being contained in the Mental Health (Care and Treatment) (Scotland) Act 2003.

Scotland also has a different form of legal system to that of the common law system of England, Northern Ireland and Wales. This is because of the influences upon the countries during the development of the law and its procedures and structures.

To add to the confusion, we are now going to use the phrase 'civil law' in a different context to the way it was described in **What is the difference between criminal and civil law? (p. 17)**. There are two main types of legal system that exist. Common law, as practised in England, Northern Ireland and Wales, and many countries with former links to England. The other type, civil law, is practised in countries that had official links to France, Germany, the Netherlands, Portugal or Spain. As we can now see, 'civil law' can be used as a type of law within a legal system, being differentiated from criminal law, or as a system of law where it is contrasted with common law.

Scotland has a mixed legal system, as it had links to both England and France during the development of its law and legal system, using elements of both common law and civil law systems in its contemporary legal system.

In keeping with healthcare practice, the law also has customs and traditions that can confuse the uninitiated. For example, in healthcare practice, once a surgeon achieves membership of the Royal College of Surgeons, it is custom that they no longer go by Dr X but become Mr or Ms X. This custom originated when surgeons undertook apprenticeships rather than university education and so were unable to use the title 'Dr'. Thus, it began as a reaction to a snub, but is now a hallmark of success.

In law, it is custom that the name of a case coming before a court follows a given formula that is distinct in criminal and civil cases. In a criminal case, the prosecution is being brought on behalf of the monarch and is generally written as R v Cornock (if I were in trouble); the R standing for Rex or Regina, king or queen, and the second part being the name of the person being prosecuted.

In a civil case, the custom uses the names of both sides, the claimant (person bringing the claim) and the defendant (person defending the claim). So, if I were to bring a claim against someone called Nichols, the case would be called Cornock v Nichols. If they sue me, the case would be called Nichols v Cornock.

This custom of naming cases allows lawyers to know who has brought the case, the first named, and who is defending it, the second named.

You may also find case names such as Re Cornock. In this instance, 'Re' means that Cornock has not brought the case but that the case is about them. It may be that the person the case concerns does not have the mental capacity to bring a case and it is being brought for their benefit/protection.

A further custom in the pronunciation of case names is worthy of note. In the names of the criminal and civil cases noted above, both parties were separated by 'v'. This is not pronounced as 'vee' or 'versus' but in a criminal case is Regina (or Rex) 'against' Cornock, whereas in a civil case, it would be Cornock 'and' Nichols.

LAW REPORTS AND THEIR ABBREVIATIONS

There are many different publishers of law reports and there is a hierarchy in terms of their use in a court case. Most of the series of law reports are referred to by abbreviations. The set of law reports highest in the hierarchy is that published by the Incorporated Council of Law Reporting since 1865 and known as The Law Reports or sometimes The *Official* Law Reports. This set of law reports has its own set of abbreviations (see table below).

To add more confusion, a system of 'neutral citations' came into being in 2001. A neutral citation is a citation for a court case given by HM Courts and Tribunals Service rather than a publisher. Neutral citations can be used to find court cases that are released directly by the HM Courts and Tribunals Service. Each neutral citation is a unique reference for a specific case and follows the format: case name [Year] court, case number starting at one each year. So, the first case in the Court of Appeal Civil Division on 2021 would be:

Nichols v Cornock [2021] EWCA civ 1

The table below shows the law report series for the abbreviations used in the case names in this book (it is in alphabetical order and not hierarchical).

Table 1.1 Law report abbreviations

Abbreviation	Law reports	Notes
AC	Appeal cases	The Law Reports
All ER	All England Law Reports	
BMLR	Butterworths Medico-Legal Reports	

Abbreviation	Law reports	Notes
Cal Rptr	California Reporter	Refers to law reports from California, United States of America
Crim LR	Criminal Law review	
ECHR	European Court of Human Rights: Reports of the Judgments and Decisions	
EWCA	Neutral citation for England and Wales Court of Appeal	Civ means Civil division Crim means Criminal division
EWHC	Neutral citation for England and Wales High Court	Ch means Chancery Division QB mean Queen's bench Division Fam means Family Division
FSR	Fleet Street Reports	
KB	King's Bench Division	The Law Reports
Lloyds Rep Med	Lloyd's Law Reports Medical	
Med LR	Medical Law Reports	
NY	New York Reports	Refers to law reports from New York, United States of America
QB	Queen's Bench Division	The Law Reports
UKHL	Neutral citation for United Kingdom House of Lords	
UKSC	Neutral citation for United Kingdom Supreme Court	
W.L.R.	Weekly Law Reports	

How do ethics and law affect me?

Ethics and law, together and separately, exist to guide your healthcare practice.

As we saw in **What are ethics? (p. 5)**, ethics comprise a way of guiding an individual's actions and behaviour for the benefit of others. In relation to healthcare, ethics are a framework which you can use when faced with dilemmas in your practice, to assist you in making a choice between two or more courses of action. By using the ethical principles discussed in **What are the main ethical principles relevant to healthcare practice? (p. 12)**, you can guide your decision making so that you consider the values that society considers to be important in your healthcare practice.

Whilst ethics are used to help determine the right outcome in a dilemma, the law has a related but different function; this is to enforce the rules that society deems to be important. To do this, the law has to state what the rule is, identify when a breach of the rule has occurred and then impose a sanction on those who have broken the rule.

Ethics and law work together for the benefit of society. Ethics outline the shared values and the law enforces these values. This is achieved though rights, duties and obligations.

As we will see in the next chapter on **Regulation (Chapter 2)**, for you, and other healthcare practitioners, ethics and law come together most notably in the way that society regulates healthcare practitioners and their practice. It is here that you will see how you are specifically affected by ethics and law. The questions in this chapter provide you with the underlying principles for that chapter and the ones that follow.

Ethics and law underpin everything you do in your practice and your relationships with your patients.

SUMMARY

- Ethics and law are vital to healthcare practice.
- Ethics are a formalised system of accepted or acceptable beliefs about how individuals within a particular group should act in a given situation.
- The law is a system of rules.
- There are several theories that provide an ethical basis for behaviour. Those traditionally used in healthcare are:
    o deontology, which is based upon duty
    o utilitarianism, the basic principle of which is that an act should be based on the premise of maximising happiness and minimising pain.
- There is no single ethical theory that applies to all healthcare dilemmas. In recognition of this, using ethical principles is a way of assisting healthcare practitioners in their ethical decision making.
- Several ethical principles are relevant to healthcare:
    o autonomy means respecting someone's ability to make decisions for themselves
    o beneficence refers to doing good
    o non-maleficence refers to not doing harm
    o justice is related to treating patients fairly, and according to their need.
- Law can arise from:
    o Acts of Parliament (statutes)
    o Common law based on judgments made in previous cases that have come before the Courts.
- There is a hierarchy of courts within the United Kingdom and judgments from the higher courts are binding (which means they have to follow them) on the lower courts.
- Law can be divided into criminal and civil law:
    o Criminal law is where a rule is deemed to be sufficiently important, the breaking of the rule is classified as a crime and is punishable by the State.
    o Civil law refers to the relationship between individuals and the mechanism by which they can settle disputes.

- The law has developed over a considerable period of time and has developed many customs that can seem arcane and confusing to the uninitiated.
- Ethics and law interact to provide a framework for healthcare practitioners so that they practise according to the shared values of society.

REFERENCES

Beauchamp, T. and Childress J. (2013) *Principles of Biomedical Ethics* (7th edition). Oxford University Press: Oxford.

Health and Care Professions Council (2016) *Standards of conduct, performance and ethics.* Health and Care Professions Council: London.

Mental Health Act 1983.

Mental Health (Care and Treatment) (Scotland) Act 2003.

Nursing and Midwifery Council (2018) *The Code.* Nursing and Midwifery Council: London.

Onions, C.T. (ed) (1984) *The Shorter Oxford English Dictionary.* Clarendon Press: Oxford.

The Health Professions Council (Registration and Fees) (Amendment) Rules Order of Council 2010 (SI 2010/479).

The Health Professions Order 2001 (SI 2002/254).

The Mental Health (Amendment) (Northern Ireland) Order 2004 (SI 2004/1272).

The Mental Health (Northern Ireland) Order 1986 (SI 1986/595).

REGULATION

Regulation affects all healthcare practitioners because it affects whether you can practise and how you ensure that you can continue to practise. Regulation may be seen as where ethics and law come together, where the ethics of society are enshrined in law for the benefit of individuals within a particular society. This chapter explores the regulation of healthcare practitioners by considering what regulation is, its purpose, how it is undertaken and the ways in which it affects the healthcare practitioner. It also discusses the concepts of responsibility, accountability and liability, and builds upon the legal and ethical framework within which healthcare practitioners have to practise.

QUESTIONS COVERED IN CHAPTER 2

- What is regulation?
- How does regulation relate to ethics and law?
- What forms of regulation exist?
- Who is the regulation of healthcare practitioners for?
- How are healthcare practitioners regulated?
- Who, or what, are healthcare regulatory bodies?
- What do the healthcare regulatory bodies do?
- What is the difference between responsibility, accountability and liability?
- As a healthcare practitioner, who am I accountable and liable to?

Q What is regulation?

A I always say, if in doubt, turn to a definition. So, *The Shorter Oxford English Dictionary* defines the verb 'regulate' as, 'to control, govern or direct by rule or regulations; to subject to guidance or restrictions … to bring or reduce a person or class of persons to order', and defines the noun 'regulation' as, 'the act of regulating, or the state of being regulated. A rule prescribed for the management of some matter, or the regulating of conduct; a governing precept or direction' (Onions, 1984).

Taking these together, we can see that regulation is concerned with rules, guidance and measures that control something, or someone, in some way, and that the control is undertaken to maintain order. If we apply this to healthcare and healthcare practitioners, it means that there is a mechanism whereby the hospitals, clinics and other areas where healthcare occurs, you and your practice are controlled.

Just before we get a little bit paranoid about being controlled, we need to acknowledge that regulation is not unique to healthcare and healthcare practitioners. Many aspects of modern life are regulated, such as food production and car safety. We also need to acknowledge that regulation is a feature of many professions and their associated practitioners; for instance, law is a regulated profession and solicitors and barristers are subject to regulation.

Indeed, for many commentators, the fact that regulation exists is a defining feature of a society because its presence indicates that there is control of aspects of the society for the benefit of its members.

For regulation to exist, there has to be something that established the mechanisms, rules, and regulations that restrict or permit an activity; an agency that oversees the act, organisation or individuals being regulated and ensures that there is compliance with the rules and guidance that are in place. For you and your fellow healthcare practitioners, this agency controls the way that you are able to go about your practice, for instance by controlling the length of your initial training period.

The control that the regulatory agency has over an activity or practitioner can be exerted in a number of ways. For instance, through the punishment of undesirable behaviour, or through rewarding behaviour that is wanted or desirable, or finally through a combination of the two. If we again turn to you and your colleagues, we can see that the healthcare practitioner who does not adhere to accepted practice, without good reason, could face a sanction by the regulatory agency, such as losing their licence to practise. Whilst those healthcare practitioners who meet the requirements of the regulatory agency are allowed to maintain their registration and thus continue in their healthcare practice.

How does regulation relate to ethics and law?

From Chapter 1 and **What is regulation? (p. 24)**, we can see that ethics and law are interwoven and that law is influenced by ethical principles. Regulation, is influenced by both ethics and law.

In this way of looking at things, regulation is a system of controls and permissions that together influence the behaviour of individuals toward behaviour that is desired.

For you, as a healthcare practitioner, the control side of regulation means that you can only practise your chosen field of healthcare if you undertake certain levels of training and education. Once you have attained these, you can then go on to practise in your chosen field, and also to expand your practice, subject to further controls; this is the permission part of regulation. By forcing you to do one thing, you are allowed to do something else.

We can now see that ethics is the first way of organising society and relies upon individuals in a society behaving according to a code of correct behaviours. Where this does not result in the desired behaviours for that society, the law steps in as the second way and punishes the unacceptable behaviour, both to correct the behaviour of the individual who has transgressed and also to warn others of what is unacceptable behaviour and to deter them from that behaviour. However, regulation as a third way, a hybrid between ethics' encouraging of 'good' behaviour and the law's punishing of unacceptable behaviours, uses a combination of restrictions and permissions that forces individuals to adopt the accepted behaviour by restricting their ability to do another thing until they do.

In order for this book to utilise a practical approach, as we progress through the questions, regulation and law will dominate our discussion. This is because both are underpinned by ethics and ethical principles. Therefore, when we discuss the law on a particular issue, we are actually discussing how society views that issue and how it wants it to be addressed; the law being the mechanism for this. When we turn to the regulation of healthcare and healthcare practitioners, we are considering the ethical and the legal principles that are underpinning the issue, and control is exerted to discourage the unwanted behaviours and permission is used to encourage wanted behaviours.

To demonstrate this, we can consider the acceptance of gifts. Let's imagine you ask, is it OK for me to accept a gift from a patient? We could answer this from any of our three approaches: ethics, law and regulation. We could go through what each of these three approaches would say, whether it is OK or not to accept a gift, and what basis they use for reaching this answer. However, do we need to consider all three approaches to reach our answer?

An ethical approach to the acceptance of a gift relates to what the gift means and the motivation of the gift giver. Is it a mark of respect and thanks or is it related to buying favour: if I give you this gift, will you give me better or preferential care? Does the patient feel obliged to provide you with a gift? Will accepting the gift compromise you or the care you give to the patient?

A legal approach would be to ask if there is anything that precludes you from accepting the gift, for example an employer policy banning the acceptance of gifts; or where the gift is given under duress, such as, if the patient believes that without the gift their care will suffer or the patient feels otherwise obliged to give the gift.

There is overlap between the first of these two approaches as the ethical principles underpin the legal approach.

Finally, we could turn to the regulatory approach with its restriction and permission. Here we would expect the regulatory agency, for you as a healthcare practitioner this will be your regulatory body (see **Who, or what, are healthcare regulatory bodies? [p. 31]**), to issue some form of rule or guidance for you to follow.

This guidance is likely to say that you cannot influence someone to give you a gift, by suggesting to the patient that their care will improve if they do or suffer if they don't. It is also likely to say that you need to follow your employer's policy, if one exists, and that gifts should only be accepted where it is given without any expectation on the part of the patient. It may even go further and say that a gift can only be accepted after a period of treatment, rather than during the treatment; in this way, the gift cannot influence the care that is being received.

This third way or regulatory approach incorporates the ethical principles relating to the meaning of the gift and motivation of the gift giver, together with the legal aspects of whether there is any prohibition on accepting a gift.

Therefore, to answer the question on whether it is OK for you to accept a gift from a patient, we would turn to the regulatory approach. In the questions that follow, we will utilise this practical approach by turning to the regulation, then the law and finally to ethics.

By the way, the answer to the question is, it depends. It depends on whether the gift is freely given (ethical approach); it depends on whether your employer has a policy in place and what the policy says (legal approach); and it depends on whether you are still treating or caring for the patient and accepting it could be seen to unbalance your practitioner–patient relationship (regulatory approach).

A final thought to consider is, how would accepting the gift look to others? Not only must you do nothing wrong, but you must be seen to be doing nothing wrong.

What forms of regulation exist?

As we will see, regulation is a form of continuum where at one end a voluntary regulatory mechanism exists and at the other end the regulation that exists is non-voluntary and imposed. Within this continuum, three core methods of regulation can be identified. These are, in order of freedom to the practitioners involved, self-regulation, state-administered regulation and state-sanctioned self-regulation.

SELF-REGULATION

Self-regulation refers to the situation where those who would be regulated appoint or elect a body to undertake the regulation, independent of any external influence. In relation to healthcare, this would mean that the regulation would be undertaken by healthcare practitioners or their chosen representatives. This could be either as a collective or as separate professions, for example nurses, physiotherapists or doctors.

There are those who see self-regulation as being a key aspect in achieving professional status, whilst others are of the opinion that healthcare, in particular medicine, was the first of the professions that was able to statutorily self-regulate.

Self-regulation gives the profession a great deal of autonomy in the way that regulation is undertaken. Genuine self-regulation is undertaken independently of any external influence, including that of the State in which it operates, for instance it would have to be free from government interference.

It can be said that there is a degree of expertise in relation to self-regulation, as it is those who practice the particular profession, and thus are those with under-standing of the practise of those being regulated, who set the limits on the actual way in which the regulation will be undertaken.

An issue with self-regulation is that it is an entirely voluntary obligation on the part of those who agree to be regulated. The accountability of the appointed or elected body is back to the members of the profession being regulated. Its very nature means that there is a lack of oversight by any external agency and the criti-cism that it is self-serving can be made.

STATE-ADMINISTERED REGULATION

At the opposite end of the continuum, state-administered regulation is a form of regulation where the regulation is undertaken by an agency of the State without any need for involvement of the profession being regulated.

In state-administered regulation, the profession has little or no role and there-fore this can be the most onerous form of regulation for a profession and its practitioners.

It can be argued that state-administered regulation is reserved for those areas where the highest risks to society and its members from poor or substandard practice exist.

STATE-SANCTIONED SELF-REGULATION

State-sanctioned self-regulation is almost at the halfway point on the regulatory continuum as it still allows the profession to be involved in the regulation process, but it is no longer voluntary for the practitioners of that profession.

Whilst the profession itself undertakes the functions of regulation, they do so under the remit and on behalf of the State. This provides the regulatory agency with the authority it needs to compel the practitioners it regulates to comply with its processes. If necessary, the State can intervene to enforce sanctions by the regulatory agency. All individuals who wish to practise in the area regulated are required to be subject to that regulation.

At present, the healthcare professions all operate under a form of state-sanctioned self-regulation.

Q Who is the regulation of healthcare practitioners for?

A This is going to come as no surprise to you but, although they are the ones who pay the fees and costs of regulation, regulation is not for the benefit of healthcare practitioners, rather it is for the protection of the public and therefore society as a whole.

One way that the public need protecting from healthcare practitioners is against those healthcare practitioners who are not competent to undertake their role; this will be explored further in the next chapter on **Duties and Standards (Chapter 3)**. Then there are those 'practitioners' who might not even be who they say they are. For instance, they may be impersonating a physiotherapist, having never undertaken a physiotherapy course or registered with the Health and Care Professions Council (see **What do the healthcare regulatory bodies do? [p. 31]**).

We would probably agree that most healthcare practitioners are conscientious individuals who are trying to do their best for their patients. However, healthcare is a partnership between the healthcare practitioner and the patient, and in any form of relationship there is the potential for an unintentional abuse of power to exist. The healthcare practitioner is most likely to be the one with the power in the relationship. This is because they are the ones who have the knowledge and skills that are required by the patient. In fact, the patient may be said to be vulnerable in this relationship.

Consider your next patient; they come to see you because they have a condition that their only knowledge of is what they have gleaned from the internet, and we know how reliable that can be! They are worried about what the condition will mean for them and their family, their lifestyle and their work. They need someone to help them. Then there is you; you know all about this condition, how it could progress and what is needed to treat it. You have all the power; the patient is helpless in terms of dealing with their condition, but you aren't.

This is another reason why healthcare practitioners are regulated. To protect patients from those healthcare practitioners who may abuse the power they can exercise over their patients. Regulation exists to balance the power dynamic in the relationship between healthcare practitioner and patient.

Reducing the possibility of errors is a further reason that healthcare practitioners are subject to regulation. By reducing errors, the public are protected from the possibility of harm that can accompany errors by healthcare practitioners. Indeed, it could be argued that healthcare practitioners should be subject to the highest form of regulation possible if this could prevent errors from occurring.

Referring to healthcare practitioners as HCPs, Cornock notes that there is a, 'particular issue relating to HCPs that does not relate to other professionals in quite the same way, [this] is that HCPs are involved in people's lives and health. The old adage is that doctors bury their mistakes. This is not as facile as it may seem. Mistakes by HCPs can, and do, result in harm to patients and ultimately their death; HCPs do not always have a second attempt to rectify an initial error' (Cornock, 2008: 34).

So, although they pay for it, regulation of healthcare practitioners exists mainly for their patients, to protect them from the incompetent, the bogus, the unsafe and the possibility of errors that may result in the patient's harm. By protecting patients, regulation protects society.

 How are healthcare practitioners regulated?

As we saw when we considered **What forms of regulation exist?** (p. 27), the current form of regulation of healthcare practitioners is by state-sanctioned self-regulation; this is undertaken by the regulatory bodies (see **Who, or what, are healthcare regulatory bodies? [p. 31]**).

The main method by which the regulatory bodies ensure the safety of the public is through the registration of individuals who are deemed competent to practise as healthcare practitioners.

We can turn to both case law and the House of Lords to support this proposition. In a 1959 case which determined if the General Nursing Council, a precursor of the current nursing regulatory body the Nursing and Midwifery Council, was a charity and thereby entitled to a reduction of its rates (it wasn't!), Lord Cohen stated, 'if I had to say which was … [the primary reason for the existence of the General Nursing Council] …, I should unhesitatingly choose the protection of the public by the provision of skilled trained nurses' (General Nursing Council for England and Wales v St Marylebone Corporation [1959]: 332). Thus, by analogy, this is the role of all healthcare practitioner regulatory bodies.

Four decades later, the House of Lords reconfirmed this position and clarified that it extended to other healthcare practitioner groups in addition to nurses, when it stated that, 'the principal purpose of regulation of any healthcare profession is to protect the public from unqualified or inadequately trained practitioners' (House of Lords Select Committee on Science and Technology, 2000: paragraph 5.1).

It could be expected that anyone who comes into contact with the patient in a healthcare setting would be subject to the same degree of regulation. However, this is not the case. The regulatory bodies only have jurisdiction over someone who is on the register that they maintain. Anyone who is not on the relevant register is not subject to discipline or sanction by the regulatory body.

In recent years, there have been calls for all those involved in healthcare practice to be subject to some form of regulatory control. However, at present, there are some individuals, who would see themselves as healthcare practitioners, who remain unregulated. For instance, although the UK Council for Psychotherapy operates as a regulator in the same way as other healthcare regulatory bodies, it is different in that registration is voluntary, leading to some psychotherapists being unregistered.

Who, or what, are healthcare regulatory bodies?

The statutory healthcare regulatory bodies, that is those where registration is compulsory for those healthcare practitioners who wish to work within the areas they regulate, are (in alphabetical order) listed in Table 2.1.

Table 2.1 Regulatory bodies

Regulatory body	Registrants
General Chiropractic Council	Chiropractors
General Dental Council	Dentists and associated healthcare practitioners, such as dental hygienists and dental nurses
General Medical Council	Doctors
General Optical Council	Optometrists and dispensing opticians
General Osteopathic Council	Osteopaths
General Pharmaceutical Council (in Northern Ireland the Pharmaceutical Society of Northern Ireland undertakes this role)	Pharmacists and pharmacy technicians
Health and Care Professions Council	Many different healthcare practitioners, including art therapists, chiropodist/podiatrists, dieticians, paramedics, operating departments practitioners, radiographers and speech and language therapists
Nursing and Midwifery Council	Midwives, nurses and nursing associates

The regulatory bodies are paid for by registrants, through the registration fee, but they can receive state money in addition. The registration fee varies enormously between the different regulatory bodies and is generally a yearly fee paid to remain on the relevant register, allowing the healthcare practitioner to continue to practise in their field.

The regulatory bodies do not act as a professional body, such as a trade union, for the healthcare practitioners they regulate. Their role is to protect the public.

Each of the regulatory bodies was established through legislation, which outlines the scope of their remit and the functions they must exercise in their pursuit of public protection.

What do the healthcare regulatory bodies do?

The regulatory bodies have, as their primary purpose, the protection of the public from healthcare practitioners unfit to practise, for example, bogus, untrained, poorly trained healthcare practitioners or those whose conduct is deemed to fall below that which is acceptable. In order to fulfil their statutory and regulatory role, the regulatory bodies all perform similar functions in relation to their registrants and those who wish to gain entry to their respective registers.

There are five main areas to the role of the regulatory bodies, which are concerned with:

- protecting entry to the register and protection of the associated titles
- education in relation to initial registration
- maintenance of clinical competence for those on the register
- producing and maintaining standards for registrants
- fitness to practise of those on the register.

Taken in combination, these five areas encompass the regulation of healthcare practitioners and are designed to protect the public.

Because the regulatory bodies operate through a system of state-sanctioned self-regulation, they need to be able to demonstrate how they operate and are themselves held to account. Ultimately, their accountability is to the public, but this is through the Privy Council, a body of advisers to the monarch, and to Parliament through the Health Select Committee.

In addition to being held to account through the mechanisms described, the healthcare regulatory bodies are themselves regulated through the Professional Standards Authority (PSA). The role of the PSA is to oversee the healthcare regulatory bodies by assessing their performance through reviews of their work and producing an annual report on each of them. Where necessary, they can also undertake a special review of a regulatory body or an aspect of their work if this is deemed to be necessary by the Secretary of State for Health and Social Care. In this way, the PSA ensures that the regulatory bodies are protecting the public in the way that they are designed to.

So how does all this affect you? Looking at each of the five areas they oversee may provide the answer.

PROTECTING ENTRY TO THE REGISTER AND PROTECTION OF THE ASSOCIATED TITLES

The regulatory bodies set the requirements for entry to their respective registers; without being registered a healthcare practitioner is unable to practise in their chosen field. As well as educational requirements, prospective registrants need to meet requirements in relation to their character and their health to gain entry to the register.

The protection of titles is the method by which the regulatory bodies protect the public from individuals who have not met their requirements for registration. They control who can use a specific title and can take action against those who fraudulently use them: it is a criminal offence to say that you are registered with a healthcare regulatory body when you are not or to dishonestly use a protected title.

One of the issues with the protection of titles is the actual titles that are protected. If a title is not protected, anyone can use it, which can be confusing and misleading for the public. For instance, 'midwife' is a protected title (The Nursing and Midwifery Order 2001, Article 44); 'nurse' is not a protected title, but 'registered nurse' is. Similarly, 'doctor' is not a protected title, but 'registered medical practitioner' is. In fact, there are some who would argue that the 'true' doctor is those in possession of a Doctor of Philosophy qualification and that medical doctors use the term 'doctor' as an honorary title. This book uses the word 'doctor' for those registered with the General Medical Council (GMC) unless there is a specific reason, such as use in legislation, to use 'registered medical practitioner'.

The Health and Care Professions Council (HCPC) has a protected title for each of the professions it regulates by virtue of Section 6(2) of the Health Professions Order 2001.

EDUCATION IN RELATION TO INITIAL REGISTRATION

As we have just seen, to register with the appropriate regulatory body, you need to fulfil certain criteria, one of which is to have completed a set programme of education with a set number of practice hours and attain stipulated competencies.

It is the regulatory bodies that set these criteria and also authorise educational institutions to provide approved programmes of study leading to registration; and undertake quality assurance checks on these programmes on a periodic basis.

MAINTENANCE OF CLINICAL COMPETENCE FOR THOSE ON THE REGISTER

It used to be that registration with a regulatory body was for life, unless you fall foul of a fitness to practise investigation. This is not the case anymore. Healthcare practitioners not only have to pay their periodic fee to maintain their registration, they also have to demonstrate that they are maintaining and developing their competence. This is generally termed 'revalidation'. It is a relatively new requirement, for instance the GMC introduced revalidation in December 2010 whilst the Nursing and Midwifery Council introduced it in April 2016.

Part of any revalidation requirement is undertaking continuing professional development (CPD). CPD is a two-part process: the first is that the healthcare practitioner has to undertake some form of learning, training or education, either formal or informal, that has relevance to their area of practice. The second part is that this needs to be recorded, and, for some regulatory body requirements, to be reflected upon so that the healthcare practitioner can show what they have learnt from the CPD and how it assists them in their practice.

PRODUCING AND MAINTAINING STANDARDS FOR REGISTRANTS

The regulatory bodies all issue their own standards or codes of conduct, for example the Nursing and Midwifery Council's (2018) *The Code* and the Health and Care Professions Council's (2016) *Standards of conduct, performance and ethics*. They have a basis in ethics and ethical principles and are designed to assist healthcare practitioners in deciding upon what is appropriate behaviour in any situation. They set out the accepted conduct of a healthcare practitioner registered with the regulatory body.

The legislation that governs the regulatory bodies provides the basis for them to issue these codes of conduct. For instance, The Medical Act 1983 (Section 35) states, 'the powers of the General Council shall include the power to provide, in such manner as the Council think fit, advice for members of the medical profession on – (a) standards of professional conduct; (b) standards of professional performance; or (c) medical ethics'; whilst The Nursing and Midwifery Order 2001, in article 3(2), states that, 'the principal functions of the Council shall be to establish from time to time standards ... conduct and performance for nurses and midwives'.

Codes of conduct may be likened to a set of regulations for the healthcare practitioner to follow. Whilst deviance from a code of conduct is not itself an unlawful act, it may be seen as evidence of misconduct on the part of a healthcare practitioner, by a court of law or a fitness to practise hearing, if they cannot provide a valid reason for their deviance from it.

FITNESS TO PRACTISE OF THOSE ON THE REGISTER

In order to assist the regulatory bodies in their protection of patients and the public, they have the ability to remove healthcare practitioners from their respective registers. This is following an investigation into the healthcare practitioner's fitness to practise.

The regulatory bodies have different, but similar, processes for determining a healthcare practitioner's fitness to practise. For example, the HCPC has a conduct and competence committee that hears complaints of misconduct and a health committee that considers whether a healthcare practitioner's practice may be impaired by a condition or illness.

The sanctions available to a regulatory body include the ability to impose the ultimate liability on your practice, that of removing you from the register and thereby preventing you from practising in your chosen profession. Other forms of sanction that the regulatory bodies can impose upon you include requiring you: to undergo training and education; to receive treatment or care for a condition before returning to practice; to work under the supervision of another registered health-care practitioner in your field; to be suspended for a period of time; or to not work in specific fields of practice or with certain groups of patients.

Q What is the difference between responsibility, accountability and liability?

A Very often when reading articles, books and even codes of conduct or standards for practice from the regulatory bodies, it can appear as though the terms 'responsibil-ity', 'accountability' and 'liability' are the same or interchangeable. Looking at definitions of 'responsibility', 'accountability' and 'liability' is not particularly help-ful in trying to determine what the differences are between them, as they are often defined in terms of each other.

Ethically, accountability and liability are usually seen as synonymous. However, legally, this is not the case and each of the terms has a very specific meaning that relates to how your practice is judged and the possible outcome that can arise as a consequence of poor practice.

Taking each of the terms in turn, we can see how they relate to you and your practice.

RESPONSIBILITY

Responsibility means to be responsible for something specific. OK, I know that's not particularly helpful to define something in terms of itself. Responsibility refers to a duty. If you are responsible for something, you are in charge of it; if it is a task, you have a duty to make sure that the task is completed.

It is as simple as that. The discharge of one's responsibility is to undertake the thing that one is responsible for. Once this has been done, there is nothing further you have to do in regards of your responsibility. The responsibility is over once the particular thing has been completed.

With responsibility, the focus is on completion of the specific task allocated to you. From this, it can be seen that responsibility is the least onerous of the terms for the healthcare practitioner.

ACCOUNTABILITY

Accountability moves beyond the mere completion of the task and adds a further element. If you are accountable for something specific, you are firstly required to do it (as you would if you were responsible for it). Once you have done this, the extra element is that you can be required to account for the way in which you undertook the task and the outcome; that is, explain or justify your actions. This is equally so if you fail to either commence or complete the task for which you are accountable.

The need to give an account is the extra element over and above the responsibility.

LIABILITY

In strict legal terms, liability means you have an obligation. It is another step in addition to the mere completion of the task. Fulfilling your duty, when you are liable for a task, requires you to firstly complete the task, to give an account of how you undertook the task (the same as with accountability) and then face the consequences of your actions.

Your account of the task and the manner in which you performed it is crucial in any further outcome under liability. For instance, if the account you give provides all the detail that is needed and satisfies those to whom you are liable, it is likely there will be no further action. On the other hand, if your account does not satisfy those to whom you are liable, there is a possibility that you can be sanctioned for either not completing the task or for the manner in which you undertook it.

From this, you will appreciate that, in general for healthcare practice, where you are said to be accountable for something, you are actually liable for it.

AN EXAMPLE

Let's assume that you have to remove some sutures from a patient's abdomen. This is something you have done many times before. As you are responsible to undertake this duty, you need to ensure that it is completed in a safe manner and that the patient is comfortable throughout. Unfortunately, somehow you manage to cut the patient whilst using the suture cutter.

Your responsibility has ended, as the sutures have been removed.

If you had accountability for the removal of the sutures, as well as completing the task, you would need to inform the patient about what happened and record the incident in the patient's notes. In addition, you could be asked to formally give an account of what happened, what went wrong and why. To who you give the account depends on who is holding you accountable, but it is likely to include your manager, who is your employer's representative.

At the point at which you have given your account, you have discharged your duty.

If, on the other hand, you had liability for the removal of the sutures, in addition to the way you would discharge your duty if you were accountable, you also have an obligation in relation to your duty. This obligation arises after you have given your account. This scenario could lead to a number of possible outcomes, including patient complaint, refresher training, employer disciplinary or investigation by the regulatory body.

 As a healthcare practitioner, who am I accountable and liable to?

In asking this question, based on what we have established in **What is the difference between responsibility, accountability and liability? (p. 35)**, we are asking who can hold you to account and who can cause you to be sanctioned in some manner.

Essentially, in the course of your healthcare practice, you are accountable and liable to anyone who you come into contact with during the course of that practice. This is because, as we will see later (see **As a healthcare practitioner, who do I have a legal duty of care to? [p. 42]**), you have a duty of care to those who your actions could affect.

You will probably not be surprised by the following list of those who you are accountable and liable to as a healthcare practitioner, in alphabetical order (because we would be unlikely to agree on an ethical or legal hierarchy, as we have different perspectives on what is paramount):

- patients
- society
- your colleagues
- your employer
- your regulatory body (if you are a registered healthcare practitioner)
- yourself.

Taking each of these in turn, let's explore how they can hold you to account and sanction your practice.

PATIENTS

A patient can hold you to account in a myriad of ways; many of which could result in your practice been sanctioned. There are a number of organisations to which a patient may make complaints about your practice. Each of these is a form of accountability in that, as part of investigating a complaint, the organisation may require you to provide your account. If your account is not deemed to be sufficient, your liability comes into play as the organisation dealing with the patient complaint decides whether or not to sanction your practice.

As well as complaints, patients are able to commence legal action in relation to the care and treatment you provided to them; this would most usually be as an action for negligence (see **What is clinical negligence?** [p. 57]).

SOCIETY

The way that society holds you accountable is through the organisations it establishes to oversee your healthcare practice. In addition, society can hold you to account through both the civil and criminal justice systems. Any action in the civil justice system would normally be through a patient's legal action (see above). If your practice is deemed to fall seriously below an acceptable standard then you may find yourself defending your practice in the criminal courts.

Another way that society can hold healthcare practitioners to account is through the media, where errant practitioners can find that they are publicly admonished: a form of 'naming and shaming'.

YOUR COLLEAGUES

Your colleagues can hold you to account both informally and formally. Informally, they may have a quiet word with you about something that hasn't gone as planned and provide suggestions as to how this can be prevented in the future; the formal route is to report you and your practice through your employer's disciplinary or patient safety processes.

Consequences that can arise are when colleagues refuse to work with you or insist that your practice is supervised.

YOUR EMPLOYER

Your employer has the right to expect you to perform your duties in a certain way and at given times. They will have issued you with a contract of employment, which states what these duties are, will outline the amount of time you are expected to work and possibly the locations where you are required to perform your duties.

If you fail to perform your duties in the way expected by your employer, they can hold you to account through their disciplinary process. They can hold you liable for your actions by suspending you from your work; placing restrictions on the extent of your practice; requiring you to work under supervision or to undertake further training before you are allowed to practise unsupervised; or ultimately, dismissing you from the position you hold.

YOUR REGULATORY BODY

The regulatory bodies have defined and published mechanisms in place to hold the healthcare practitioners on their registers to account. This is one of the key mechanisms by which they protect the public and ensure patient safety.

For detail on this, see **What do the healthcare regulatory bodies do? (p. 31).**

YOURSELF

If any part of the list surprised you, it was probably seeing that you can hold yourself accountable and liable for your actions as a healthcare practitioner. This is not a legal or formal ethical liability. Yet, you should be your greatest critic. It is you who decides upon your level of competence and you who therefore ultimately makes the decision on whether you will offer a particular treatment to a particular patient at a particular point in time.

Because of this, you should regularly reflect and review your practice in order that you can learn from both what has gone well, as well as noting areas for improvement. By doing this, you are in effect holding yourself to account. With regard to the liability aspect, if you ever felt that you were not competent to undertake a particular treatment, you should not do so; this is a form of regulating your own practice. Indeed, it can be said to be the hallmark of the highest level of practice, as it ensures that patients only receive the care and treatment that you feel you are competent to provide.

If you do not hold yourself to account, it is you who has to live with the consequences of your actions.

SUMMARY

- At its simplest, regulation may be seen as the act of regulating; that is, the act of controlling and keeping in order through the use of rules and guidance.
- Regulation can be seen as a third way, along with ethics and law, as a system of organisation: a system of controls and permissions that together influence the behaviour of individuals.
- Three main forms of regulation can be identified: self-regulation by a profession; state-sanctioned self-regulation; and state-administered regulation. Healthcare practitioners are currently subject to state-sanctioned self-regulation.
- In the main, regulation exists to protect patients and society from those healthcare practitioners who are not fit to practise.
- Healthcare practitioners are regulated through the regulatory bodies.
- There are different statutory regulatory bodies for different healthcare practitioners. They exist to protect the public and are paid for by the registration fees of their registrants.

- The regulatory bodies protect the public through five main mechanisms, including maintaining a register of healthcare practitioners entitled to practise and assessing the fitness to practise of those registrants where a concern has been raised.
- Responsibility, accountability and liability are not synonymous in a legal context and have distinct meanings. An individual is responsible for their actions; is accountable to explain their actions; and is liable for the consequences of their actions.
- Healthcare practitioners are accountable and liable to their patients; the society in which they live and practise; their regulatory body, if they are registered with one; their colleagues; their employer; and themselves.

REFERENCES

Cornock, M. (2008) *Regulation and Control of Health Care Professionals*. Unpublished PhD thesis: Cardiff University.

General Nursing Council for England and Wales v St Marylebone Corporation [1959] 1 All ER 325.

Health and Care Professions Council (2016) *Standards of conduct, performance and ethics*. Health and Care Professions Council: London.

House of Lords Select Committee on Science and Technology (2000) *Report on Complementary and Alternative Medicine*. The Stationery Office: London.

Medical Act 1983.

Nursing and Midwifery Council (2018) *The Code*. Nursing and Midwifery Council: London.

Onions, C.T. (ed) (1984) *The Shorter Oxford English Dictionary*. Clarendon Press: Oxford.

The Health Professions Order 2001 (SI 2002/254).

The Nursing and Midwifery Order 2001 (SI 2002/253).

DUTIES AND STANDARDS

Healthcare practitioners have duties that they are required to meet and in meeting them they have to ensure that they reach a minimum standard. In this chapter, we explore what it means to have a legal duty and who a healthcare practitioner has a legal duty to. We also consider to what standard the healthcare practitioner has to perform their practice and what the possible consequences of failing to meet the required standard could be. Through the relationship between these duties and the standards that have to be met, we can see how ethics and law interplay to create an environment within which healthcare is practised, where patients are protected against poor practice and healthcare practitioners know what is expected of them.

QUESTIONS COVERED IN CHAPTER 3

- As a healthcare practitioner, who do I have a legal duty of care to?
- Do I have a duty to individuals outside my clinical practice?
- What is the legal standard I have to reach in my practice?
- Do I have to treat or care for a challenging patient if I feel that doing so may put me in physical danger?
- Are trainee and student healthcare practitioners held to the same standard as a registered healthcare practitioner?
- Does the standard of care change if you undertake advanced practice or work in an advanced role?
- How does delegation affect liability?
- I work as part of a team; if I follow someone else's order then are they at fault if something goes wrong and not me?
- What should I do if I am concerned about the actions of a colleague?
- What is evidence-based practice and how does it relate to my practice?
- How up to date do I need to be?
- Can I be sued in the execution of my duties?
- What is clinical negligence?
- What is the duty of candour?
- Is it OK to say sorry?
- What is vicarious liability?
- Do I need an indemnity arrangement?

Q As a healthcare practitioner, who do I have a legal duty of care to?

A A legal duty of care is an obligation placed on an individual which requires them to act in a certain way, and to a given standard, towards others to avoid harming them. The duty of care is often referred to as having liability for one's actions.

Most people would agree that if a healthcare practitioner was caring for or treating a patient, they would have a duty of care towards that patient. So far so clear! You have a legal duty of care to your patients. However, is this the extent of your duty of care, or does it extend further?

As you might expect, your duty of care extends beyond the patient immediately in front of you.

The legal principle of when a duty of care is owed was established in 1932 in a case involving a bottle of ginger beer and a snail.

CASE NOTE 3.1

DONOGHUE V STEVENSON [1932]

Mrs Donoghue and a friend went into a café where the friend bought two drinks. Mrs Donoghue's drink was ginger beer served in an opaque bottle. Some of this was poured into a glass which Mrs Donoghue drank. Later, the rest of the ginger beer was poured from the bottle into the glass and, what was said to be, a decomposed snail came out of the bottle. Mrs Donoghue was said to suffer shock and gastric illness as a consequence of drinking the ginger beer.

Mrs Donoghue wanted to take action for the shock and gastric illness she had suffered. However, she had not paid for the ginger beer and so had no contract with the manufacturer or the café owner. This left her without any apparent recourse to legal action and so she sought a decision from the Courts as to whether there was a course of action open to her in seeking damages from the manufacturer.

The case went through the legal system to the House of Lords where it was decided that a manufacturer had a duty to take reasonable care to the ultimate consumer of their product, even if there was no contract between the two parties.

The Donoghue case established what has become known as the 'neighbour principle' as the legal principle of deciding if a duty of care exists. It is known as the 'neighbour principle' because, when outlining the basis for deciding if a duty of care exists between individuals, Lord Atkin stated that, 'you must take reasonable care to avoid acts or omissions which you can reasonably foresee would be likely to injure your neighbour' (Donoghue v Stevenson [1932]: 580).

Lord Atkin then went on to address what this neighbour principle entails, stating: 'Who then, in law, is my neighbour? The answer seems to be persons who are so closely and directly affected by my act that I ought reasonably to have them in my contemplation as being so affected when I am directing my mind to the acts or omissions which are called in question' (Donoghue v Stevenson [1932]: 580).

The 'neighbour principle' means that when you are considering undertaking an act you need to also consider who could be affected by that act and take reasonable steps to ensure that you do not harm those individuals in your performance of that act.

The 'neighbour principle' is over 85 years old and has been restated in subsequent legal cases but not radically altered. The legal basis for establishing whether a health-care practitioner has a duty of care to another individual is that of proximity.

From a legal perspective, proximity relates to having the other person in mind when you undertake an action. Following the judgment in a case where someone tried to sue an auditor for misreporting financial accounts (Caparo Industries PLC v Dickman and others [1990]), to determine whether a duty is owed, it is necessary to consider whether the following factors exist:

- reasonable foresight of harm
- sufficient proximity of relationship
- that it is fair, just and reasonable to impose a duty.

The first two factors relate to the 'neighbour principle', whilst the third factor, arising from the Caparo Industries case, allows the court to consider whether establishing a duty in certain circumstances would impose too onerous a duty on individuals.

In deciding whether a duty of care was owed to a particular individual, a judge would use a two-stage test. The first stage is the law stage and asks whether the particular circumstances of the case are capable of resulting in a duty of care by the healthcare practitioner to the individual; this is based on the application of the 'neighbour principle'. The second stage is the factual stage and asks whether, in the facts of the case, one party owed the other a duty of care.

These are situations where the court accepts that a duty of care is capable of existing between individuals who have a special relationship between each other, without the need to prove that a duty of care existed. This is in so-called 'established duty situations'. Examples of this include between healthcare practitioners and their patients, or between employer and employee. Therefore, if a patient were to bring a clinical negligence claim against a healthcare practitioner, they would not need to prove that this is the sort of situation where a duty of care can exist (the law stage). They would still have to prove the factual stage, that is, whether the specific healthcare practitioner owed a duty of care to them in the circumstances of the case.

Within healthcare, the legal position is that a duty of care is owed to any patient or client of a National Health Service (NHS) Trust or organisation. Any employee or contractor of a NHS Trust or organisation, including healthcare practitioners and support staff such as porters and administration staff, will have a duty of care to each and every patient or client. The precise nature of the duty of care by a healthcare practitioner will be dependent upon their relationship with the patient or client.

Both within the NHS and in independent settings, where a healthcare practitioner has a clinical relationship with a patient, it is considered that they have an established duty of care to that patient. Essentially, the duty of care exists when the healthcare practitioner takes responsibility for any aspect of the patient's clinical needs.

Healthcare practitioners have to abide by the same duty of care principles as anyone else, therefore the 'neighbour principle' applies to you and you have a duty to anyone who is or may be affected by your actions or omissions.

Given that your actions may also affect your colleagues, the relatives of patients, your employer, and other individuals who are in the vicinity of you undertaking your practice, by applying the 'neighbour principle', you have a duty of care to these people.

Summary of when you have a duty of care to patients:

- If you touch a patient – you have a duty.
- If you are assigned a patient – you have a duty.
- If the patient is in the care of your employer – you have a duty.
- If you have an independent contract to provide care to a patient – you have a duty.

Q Do I have a duty to individuals outside my clinical practice?

A Commonly, providing care outside of the work environment is referred to as the act of a 'Good Samaritan'.

There is no 'Good Samaritan' law in the United Kingdom at present. However, the principle was considered in the case of Ms F and whether she could be sterilised.

CASE NOTE 3.2

F V WEST BERKSHIRE HEALTH AUTHORITY [1989]

This case concerned a 36-year-old woman who suffered from a serious mental disability, which meant she had the mental capacity of a 4-year-old child. She was an in-patient at a hospital and had formed a sexual relationship with another patient. It was felt that it would not be in F's best interests to get pregnant.

The case was about whether it would be lawful to sterilise F given that she was unable to give consent on her own behalf because of her lack of capacity to do so.

It was decided that it would be lawful to perform the sterilisation because it was in the best interests of F.

As part of the judgment, the Law Lords hearing the case considered the position of someone acting outside of their duty to care. Lord Goff stated: 'The "doctor in the house" who volunteers to assist a lady in the audience who, overcome by the drama or by the heat in the theatre, has fainted away is impelled to act by no greater duty than that imposed by his own Hippocratic Oath' (F v West Berkshire Health Authority [1989]: 567).

This case illustrates that a case that concerns one thing, sterilisation of a patient lacking capacity, can have an outcome on another aspect of healthcare practice, the duty to act outside of the clinical environment.

As we can clearly see from Ms F's case, although Lord Goff was speaking about doctors, the same legal point applies to all healthcare practitioners – there is no legal obligation upon you to act in an emergency outside of your work environment, for instance at the scene of an accident, where you are not on duty.

The only obligation would be where the person in need of attention was an existing patient of the healthcare practitioner. In this situation, there is likely to be an existing duty to act.

However, as Lord Goff notes, although there is no legal duty to act, there may be an ethical duty upon you to act in an emergency (see **What are the traditional ethical theories for healthcare? [p. 6]**). It can be argued that the healthcare practitioner's codes of conduct, for instance those issued by the Health and Care Professions Council (HCPC) or Nursing and Midwifery Council (NMC), place a requirement upon the healthcare practitioner to act in an emergency; although this is not always explicitly stated in the codes. For instance, the NMC code states, 'Always offer help if an emergency arises in your practice setting or anywhere else' (Nursing and Midwifery Council, 2018: paragraph 15), which is quite clear about the need to act outside of the work environment. However, the HCPC code does not say anything explicit about acting outside of the work environment but does state, 'You must make sure that your conduct justifies the public's trust and confidence in you and your profession' (Health and Care Professions Council, 2016: paragraph 9.1), which is less clear but can be interpreted that, if the public would expect you to act in an emergency in the street and you don't, you would not be justifying their trust.

Where no pre-existing duty of care exists and you decide to assist a member of the public, you are assuming a duty of care to that person. You will then be subject to all the legal principles relating to treating a patient, for instance meeting the required standard of care. This has prohibited some healthcare practitioners from wanting to assist in emergencies.

In recognition of the fact that healthcare practitioners, and others, who assisted in an emergency potentially faced being sued for negligence if something went wrong, the government introduced the Social Action, Responsibility and Heroism Act 2015. This Act requires the court to consider whether a person acting in an emergency was acting in the public interest and, if so, whether it is reasonable to allow a claim in negligence to succeed against them. It essentially extends the principle of whether it is fair, just and reasonable to impose a duty (see **As a healthcare practitioner, who do I have a legal duty of care to? [p. 42]**) to situations where the person assumes a duty of care. It means that those assuming a duty of care that benefits the public have a degree of protection against being sued for negligence.

Q What is the legal standard I have to reach in my practice?

A If a healthcare practitioner owes a duty of care to their patient and does not meet the necessary standard, from a legal perspective, the duty of care is said to have been breached.

Over the years, a number of standards have been used in the Courts to judge whether the legal duty of care has been met or breached; each standard building upon the last.

In 1932, the concept of 'the man on the Clapham Omnibus' as a representative of the common or ordinary man was proposed as being an independent arbitrator of what an acceptable standard is in a given situation. As Lord Justice Greer states in Hall v Brooklands Auto-Racing Club [1932] (a case involving a spectator injured during a crash at a motor racing event), the standard, 'must be judged by what any reasonable member of the public must have intended should be the terms of the contract. The person concerned is sometimes described as "the man in the street", or "the man on the Clapham Omnibus"' (Hall v Brooklands Auto-Racing Club [1932]: 217).

'The man on the Clapham Omnibus" was the reasonable ordinary person who could apply their commonsense to a given situation to determine what standard should be applied to a duty of care to determine if the duty was met or breached. In essence, the standard was what would a reasonable person expect you to do to meet your duty of care.

This was all well and good where the 'the man on the Clapham Omnibus' was able to understand the complexities of the duty of care in any particular set of circumstances. However, where special skill is involved in meeting the duty of care, it may be that, rather than the reasonable ordinary 'man on the Clapham Omnibus', someone with knowledge of the special skills and abilities was needed to judge the duty and determine if the standard was met or breached.

Within the legal system, a more objective and precise standard than that of the 'man on the Clapham Omnibus' evolved where a special skill is involved in meeting a duty of care. The standard that has resulted is that of the 'Bolam test', which originated from a case concerning an allegation of clinical negligence.

CASE NOTE 3.3

BOLAM V FRIERN HOSPITAL MANAGEMENT COMMITTEE [1957]

The patient, Mr Bolam, was admitted to hospital for electroconvulsive therapy. He agreed to the treatment and signed a consent form. However, he was not warned that a possible complication of the treatment was one or more fractures. Mr Bolam received his electroconvulsive therapy successfully on the first occasion but, on the second, did in fact suffer some fractures.

Neither Mr Bolam nor the hospital disputed that the use of relaxant drugs would have prevented the risk of fractures occurring. At the time Mr Bolam received his treatment, there were two schools of opinion as to the use of relaxant drugs: one that they should be used to prevent fractures, the other that there was risk involved with the use of relaxants and they should only be used where there were particular indicators for their use and instead manual restraint should be used. Mr Bolam had received manual restraint instead of relaxant drugs.

Mr Bolam sued his consultant for breaching the duty of care owed to him by not using relaxant drugs. Mr Bolam lost his case as it was held that, as there were two bodies of opinion regarding the use of relaxant drugs, the consultant had met his duty of care by following one of the bodies of opinion.

In the case, Mr Justice McNair noted that, 'Where you get a situation which involves the use of some special skill or competence, then the test whether there has been negligence [breach of the duty of care] or not is not the test of the man on the Clapham Omnibus, because he has not got this special skill. The test is the standard of the ordinary skilled man exercising and professing to have that special skill. A man need not possess the highest expert skill at the risk of being found negligent. It is well established law that it is sufficient if he exercises the ordinary skill of an ordinary competent man exercising that particular art' (Bolam v Friern Hospital Management Committee [1957]: 121).

What Mr Justice McNair is saying is that the standard of care that has to be met is, what a responsible body of other healthcare practitioners with the same skills and knowledge as you would do in the same circumstances; you are in effect being held to a standard set by the actions of your peers. This is the 'Bolam test' or standard that has to be met.

Since the adoption of the 'Bolam test', there have been concerns that, although the matter as to whether a duty of care exists is a legal question and the standard of care test has been set through common law, the actual standard of care in any given case is not an objective test but a matter of professional judgement. This has led to some commentators concluding that healthcare practitioners are judged by their colleagues rather than by the Courts.

In negligence cases heard by the Courts, expert witnesses are called by both sides to provide evidence as to whether the practice by the healthcare practitioner in question is one that a responsible body of practitioners would have undertaken in the same circumstances. This has led to situations where judges have had to choose the opinion of one expert witness rather than the other. Lord Scarman noted that this was not an acceptable practice; in Maynard v West Midlands Regional Health Authority [1984], a case which concerned whether an exploratory operation for Hodgkin's disease should have been delayed until the outcome of a test for tuberculosis was known, he stated that, 'A judge's "preference" for one body of distinguished professional opinion to another also professionally distinguished is not sufficient to establish negligence in a practitioner whose actions have received the seal of approval of those whose opinions, truthfully expressed, honestly held, were not preferred. If this was the real reason for the judge's finding, he erred in law even though elsewhere in his judgment he stated the law correctly. For in the realm of diagnosis and treatment negligence is not established by preferring one respectable body of professional opinion to another. Failure to exercise the ordinary skill of a doctor (in the appropriate speciality, if he be a specialist) is necessary' (Maynard v West Midlands Regional Health Authority [1984]: 639).

This led to the situation in the case of Patrick Bolitho where a judge concluded that, although both sides presented their own expert opinion, the view put forward by the defendant's expert witnesses was not logical or sensible. However, by application of the 'Bolam test', the evidence of a responsible body of healthcare practitioner is sufficient to meet the standard requirement, therefore anyone following this standard would not be judged to have breached the required duty of care, even where it is not logical.

CASE NOTE 3.4

BOLITHO V CITY AND HACKNEY HEALTH AUTHORITY [1998]

This case concerned the death of 2-year-old Patrick Bolitho. Patrick had suffered with croup and been discharged from hospital, but needed to be readmitted as he was suffering breathing difficulties, and later died. A case of negligence, failing to meet the duty of care, was brought against the consultant. It was agreed by both parties that a duty of care was owed to Patrick by the consultant. It was also agreed that, had Patrick been intubated, he would not have suffered respiratory failure and cardiac arrest. The failure of the consultant to see Patrick on three occasions when he had respiratory difficulties was found to be a breach of duty; however, the issue related to the actions which the consultant could have taken had he seen Patrick.

Utilising the 'Bolam test', the case centred on whether the consultant would have intubated Patrick on assessing him. There was a body of responsible opinion that would not have intubated Patrick. The consultant acted in accordance with this opinion and so it was held that the breach in not seeing Patrick had not caused his death.

In the appeal of the case to the House of Lords, Lord Browne-Wilkinson declared that,

A court is not bound to hold that a doctor can escape liability for negligence merely by producing evidence from a number of experts that his opinion accorded with medical practice. The body of opinion relied upon must have a basis in logic, and the judge must be satisfied that the experts have directed their minds to the question of comparative risks and benefits and have reached a defensible conclusion on the matter (Bolitho v City and Hackney Health Authority [1998]: 242).

This advances the 'Bolam test' in that any opinion put forward must now be reasonable, logical and capable of withstanding examination; what has become known as the 'Bolitho test'. This has not replaced the 'Bolam test' but modified it so that the standard of care required of a healthcare practitioner in meeting their duty of care may now be stated as:

> A healthcare practitioner must reach the standard of the ordinary competent practitioner professing to have the skills and knowledge required to undertake the specific action performed, and this standard must be capable of withstanding logical scrutiny.

It is no longer possible to say that you have met your duty of care because you have done what someone else says they would have done in the same circumstances, if that person cannot provide a logical basis for their actions. This moves the 'Bolam test' from being a purely professional opinion to a more objective test.

Q **Do I have to treat or care for a challenging patient if I feel that doing so may put me in physical danger?**

A It will probably come as no surprise to you to learn that you have a duty of care to all patients that you come into contact with, but that how you discharge that duty varies. It will also not be a surprise that your actions will be judged using the 'Bolam test' (see **What is the legal standard I have to reach in my practice? [p. 46]**).

Patients can be challenging for a number of reasons. A patient who appears drunk may not understand the care they are being given; whilst the aggressive patient may be resisting treatment altogether. However, the 'drunken patient' may be suffering from a condition, such as ataxia or having diabetes and a low blood sugar level, that causes them to be unsteady and appear drunk. Likewise, a patient who is being aggressive may have a low blood oxygen level or is frightened and/or unable to understand what is happening.

Because aggression and violence may be the result of an underlying illness and certain illnesses can be mistaken for the patient being drunk, there is an expectation that you would try to ascertain the underlying problem, in so far as you can gain the patient's co-operation. Therefore, you still have a duty of care to the aggressive or drunk patient and will be expected to discharge your duty to the same standard that another healthcare practitioner would.

However, it is important to remember that you do not have to put yourself at risk in the discharge of your duty. You are only expected to meet the standard of the reasonable body of your peers (the 'Bolam test') and not a superhero who puts themselves at risk in discharging their duty. By this I mean that you do not have to risk personal injury to treat or care for a patient. You should take reasonable steps to assist the patient but, where there is a risk of physical danger to you or others, you are entitled to request assistance and to withdraw to safety until that assistance arrives.

There is also a duty on your employer to have a system in place for dealing with aggressive or violent patients. This should include training for you and a way of summoning assistance when you need it.

Are trainee and student healthcare practitioners held to the same standard as a registered healthcare practitioner?

Unfortunately for trainee healthcare practitioners, there is a strong body of common law which states that learners and juniors have to achieve the same standard as their more senior registered or qualified colleagues.

In 1952, Lord Justice Denning concluded that, 'errors due to inexperience or lack of supervision are no defence against the injured person' (Jones v Manchester Corporation [1952]: 871, which involved a patient dying as a result of the combination of drugs that were administered to him). In a later case, which was concerned with the alleged negligence of a learner driver, it was held that a, 'driver, however inexperienced and whatever his disabilities, owed the same standard of care [as a competent and experienced driver] to any passenger in the car, including an instructor, for to hold otherwise would lead to varying standards applicable to different drivers and hence to endless confusion and injustice' (Nettleship v Weston [1971]: 582).

Thus, there is a general legal principle that learners and inexperienced individuals need to meet the same standard as that of their more experienced colleagues. This principle was considered in relation to learner and inexperienced healthcare practitioners in the Wilsher case.

CASE NOTE 3.5

WILSHER V ESSEX AREA HEALTH AUTHORITY [1986]

The key aspects of this case concern a prematurely born baby who needed oxygen to be administered. In order to monitor the amount of oxygen being administered, an arterial catheter was needed. This was inserted by an inexperienced doctor who asked the registrar to check the placement of the catheter. When checking the catheter, the registrar failed to notice that it was placed in a vein and not an artery. Additionally, when the catheter needing replacing, the registrar also inserted it into a vein. As a result of responding to erroneous blood values, the infant received too much oxygen.

The baby was later diagnosed with an incurable retinal condition that limited his vision. One of the five possible causes of this retinal condition was the excess of oxygen administered. As such, the mother, who brought the case against the hospital and doctors, was unable to establish which of the five possible causes was the actual cause of the baby's retinal condition.

One of the key aspects of the Wilsher case was whether both the doctors, the inexperienced junior who wrongly sited the catheter and the registrar who failed to notice the incorrect placement, had met their duty of care to the baby. In the case, Lord Justice Glidewell stated that, 'In my view, the law requires the trainee or learner to be judged by the same standard as his more experienced colleagues. If he did not, inexperience would frequently be urged as a defence to an action for professional negligence' (Wilsher v Essex Area Health Authority [1986]: 831).

This means that both the inexperienced junior doctor and the registrar had to meet the same standard to meet their duty of care to the baby.

For those of you who consider that Lord Justice Glidewell, and indeed the law, is being unsympathetic or insensitive to the needs of learners and the inexperienced healthcare practitioner, consider what else Lord Justice Glidewell has to say: 'I should add that, in my view, the inexperienced doctor called on to exercise a specialist skill will, as part of that skill, seek the advice and help of his superiors when he does or may need it. If he does seek such help, he will have satisfied the test, even though he may himself have made a mistake' (Wilsher v Essex Area Health Authority [1986]: 831).

Lord Justice Glidewell, and the law itself, is acknowledging that learners and inexperienced members of the team do not have to achieve the same level of competence as that of the more experienced healthcare practitioner. However, they do have to achieve the same standard as their more experienced colleagues. The standard is that of the 'Bolam test' (see **What is the legal standard I have to reach in my practice? [p. 46]**). This is an important distinction; the standard is the same, but the competence shown in achieving that standard is different.

What this means is that both doctors in the Wilsher case had to meet the 'Bolam test' as the standard of their duty of care. Taking the facts of the case, the inexperienced doctor had to do what other inexperienced doctors would do, seek the advice of their more senior and experienced colleagues, which the doctor in the Wilsher v Essex Area Health Authority [1986] case did. The registrar on the other hand had to meet the standard of other registrars, who it could be said would not have missed the placement of the catheter in the vein rather than the artery or would not have inserted a catheter into a vein themselves without noticing this. On this basis, the inexperienced doctor met their duty of care whilst the registrar did not.

Thus, all those involved in healthcare delivery are judged against the standard of the 'Bolam test', that is by what a responsible body of their peers would do in the same circumstances. However, the trainee, learner or inexperienced healthcare practitioner may meet the standard of the 'Bolam test' by doing what others who are inexperienced would do: by acknowledging their inexperience and asking a more experienced colleague for advice or guidance.

Does the standard of care change if you undertake advanced practice or work in an advanced role?

The standard of care remains the same regardless of your level within the hierarchy, or the specific role that you undertake. The way that you will meet the standard also remains the same. What does change is the level of competence you will need to demonstrate in meeting the standard.

The standard for any healthcare practitioner is that of the 'Bolam test' as modified by the principles of the 'Bolitho test' (see **What is the legal standard I have to reach in my practice? [p. 46]**); that is, by comparison with a responsible body of your peers and what they would do in the same circumstances, as long as it is logical. However, if you act outside of your normal role, by taking on what used to be called an 'extended role', or you undertake advanced practice, that is practice not normally undertaken by those at your level, you will be compared to those who normally undertake those roles. This means that the 'Bolam test' still applies but the peer group changes from your normal peer group to the group of people who profess to have the skill that you are practising.

For instance, if you were to undertake roles normally undertaken by a doctor, when the 'Bolam test' is applied to your practice, the responsible body of opinion will be provided by doctors and not your professional group. Likewise, if you are newly registered and take on roles that are normally practised by advanced practitioners, you will be judged against those advanced practitioners rather than other newly-registered practitioners.

With regard to advanced practitioners, that is those who are working at a level beyond that normally expected for their role, the words of Lord Scarman are relevant; he said that, 'a doctor who professes to exercise a special skill must exercise the ordinary skill of his speciality' (Maynard v West Midlands Regional Health Authority [1984]: 638), and see **What is the legal standard I have to reach in my practice? (p. 46)**. What he is saying is that if you claim to have a skill that is above that normally possessed by those in your role or grade, you must carry out that skill in the same way that others who normally undertake the practice of that skill do. You do not have to reach the pinnacle of perfection in practising that skill, but equally you cannot compare yourself to how someone who does not have that skill will perform it.

Similarly, if a learner healthcare practitioner was to go beyond their role and undertake practice that is only undertaken by a registered healthcare practitioner, they will be judged against registered healthcare practitioners in determining whether they have breached the standard of care rather than other learners.

If you work outside of your level of competence to meet the standard required by the 'Bolam test', you are not judged against the skills and competence you have, but rather what you should have to undertake that role and you are compared to those who normally undertake that role.

The key point here is to work within your level of competence.

Q How does delegation affect liability?

A Every healthcare practitioner, from the most junior or inexperienced to the most senior, is liable for their own actions (see **As a healthcare practitioner, who do I have a legal duty of care to?** [p. 42]). This means that, if something goes wrong, they will have to account for their own actions, and personally face the consequences of these actions. If one healthcare practitioner delegates a task to another and asks them to do something that they are not competent to do, if anything were to go wrong, both healthcare practitioners will be liable for their own actions; the one who delegated for inappropriate delegation and the one who was delegated to for taking on a task that they were not competent to do.

The reason for this is that, although the task has been delegated to them, the healthcare practitioner is liable for the manner in which they undertake that task; and the delegator should ensure that they only delegate tasks to those who are competent to undertake them. Having a task delegated to you, or following someone else's orders, does not absolve you from legal liability.

Best practice would be not to take on a task that you are not competent to do and not to delegate to someone without checking that they are competent to undertake the task.

Q I work as part of a team; if I follow someone else's order then are they at fault if something goes wrong and not me?

A Whilst some healthcare practitioners believe that working as part of a team means that they have no individual liability, there is no concept of team liability in law. Therefore, working as part of a team does not absolve you from personal legal liability.

Each member of a healthcare team will have liability for their actions as part of that team. If an untoward event were to occur, it would not be the team as a whole that would be held liable but the individual member or members of the team that were deemed to be responsible, with each being liable for their own individual actions in relation to the incident. Likewise, the person in charge of the team or the person leading the team would not assume liability for all team members, or for the actions of the team, but would be liable for their own part in relation to the event.

As we saw when considering **What is the legal standard I have to reach in my practice?** (p. 46), the standard to which each member of the multidisciplinary healthcare team is judged is that of the 'Bolam test'. The standard is one where the healthcare practitioner is compared to a responsible body of their peers and what they would do in the same circumstances.

Although each member of the healthcare team is judged against the same standard, that of the 'Bolam test', they do not have to achieve the same level of competence. Lord Justice Mustill made this principle clear when he stated that, if the law, 'seeks to attribute to each individual member of the team a duty to live up to the standards demanded of the unit [team] as a whole, it cannot be right, for it would expose a student nurse to an action in negligence for a failure to possess the skill and experience of a consultant' (Wilsher v Essex Area Health Authority [1986]: 813; see **Are trainee and student healthcare practitioners held to the same standard as a registered healthcare practitioner? [p. 50]**). So, although each member of the team is held to the same standard, the 'Bolam test', the way they have to meet that test is different and related to their own area of practice and level of competence.

Therefore, if the healthcare team in question comprised nurses and doctors, although each individual member of the team would be judged against the 'Bolam test', each would be judged by the standards of their own professional group; the nurse by fellow nurses and the doctor by fellow doctors. There are exceptions to this, for example when a nurse assumes the role usually taken by a doctor which is considered in detail in **Does the standard of care change if you undertake advanced practice or work in an advanced role? (p. 52)**.

As a part of multidisciplinary team working, a healthcare practitioner may have a task delegated to them. As we saw when we deliberated **How does delegation affect liability? (p. 53)**, the fact that a task is delegated to them does not absolve a healthcare practitioner from their liability for that task.

What should I do if I am concerned about the actions of a colleague?

Raising a concern about a colleague can be a difficult and uncomfortable experience. However, where the actions or behaviour of a colleague give rise to concern, it is the duty of a healthcare practitioner to promote and uphold patient safety and this encompasses the need to put the patient before working relationships. For those healthcare practitioners registered with a regulatory body, this is enshrined within the regulatory body's codes of conduct.

When raising a concern, it is important that it is raised with the appropriate individual or authority. Employers and organisations, such as universities for those in training, are expected to have a policy that details how to raise a concern and the process for doing so. In most cases, this would initially be your line manager. Ideally your line manager will be able to act on your concern and bring it to the attention of the line manager of the colleague you have the concern about. If this is not possible then they should raise it with their line manager for them to act upon it.

Where you are unable to raise your concern with your line manager, you should consult your employer's policy to see whether there is a designated individual or 'office' where concerns can be raised.

If your line manager or the designated individual deals with your concern to your satisfaction, this should be the end of the issue. However, if you are not satisfied with the outcome of your concern or the way it has been dealt with, you can escalate your concern according to the process in your employer's policy. This may be to the senior healthcare practitioner for your profession, the head of department or a specific member of the organisation's management team.

If your concern is still not dealt with satisfactorily or you are unable to raise it internally, you should consider raising it with the regulatory body of healthcare practitioner you have concerns about, or one of the quality assurance agencies such as the Care Quality Commission.

Taking a concern externally is usually referred to as 'whistleblowing' and it is important that you raise any concern you have with an appropriate authority which can take action. You must avoid raising it with organisations that are unable to act on your concern, such as the media.

There is protection in place for whistleblowers who act in good faith, follow the appropriate process and have a reasonable belief that they are acting in the public interest, for instance protecting individuals from harm. This is through the Public Interest Disclosure Act 1998 which protects whistleblowers from being treated unfairly in relation to the raising of their concern.

If you belong to one, you may want to seek advice from a professional organisation, trade union or an indemnity provider before raising a concern, especially before taking a concern external to your organisation.

It is good practice to make a record of the concerns you have raised, including the dates and times of when you raised them and with whom.

What is evidence-based practice and how does it relate to my practice?

How do you know that the care and treatment you give to your patients is the correct care and treatment for their needs? Presumably you will base your treatment decisions on your experience of having treated the condition previously, your knowledge of the condition and the available treatment and information from colleagues. You will be using the evidence you have from these different sources in making your treatment decisions. That is, you will be basing your practice upon the evidence available to you, and by doing so you have demonstrated evidence-based practice (EBP).

As a consequence of the Bolitho case (see **What is the legal standard I have to reach in my practice? [p. 46]**), any decision made by a healthcare practitioner has to have a rational basis and withstand logically scrutiny. Thus, the Bolitho case can be said to be responsible, indirectly, for the upsurge in interest in EBP that occurred after the judgment in the case. Although it is equally true to say that the healthcare failures in the 1990s and early 2000s, such as that of the paediatric cardiac services at the Bristol Royal Infirmary, brought EBP into mainstream healthcare practice.

If there is no evidence base to support a decision that a healthcare practitioner has made, do they meet the standard required by the 'Bolam test'? It is almost impossible for them to do so, as part of the 'Bolam test' now includes the test introduced by the Bolitho case.

From the Bolitho case onwards, in order to demonstrate a rational basis for their decision making in practice, healthcare practitioners needed to be able to point to the evidence that they used to support their clinical decision making.

An example of evidence that can be used to support a decision is the use of guidelines, such as those from the National Institute for Health and Care Excellence (NICE). It is not just using a guideline that is important. The healthcare practitioner will need to show why the specific guideline they referred to was appropriate for that patient and that the guideline was the most recent version they could be expected to know about. If a healthcare practitioner decides not to follow a guideline, they would need to demonstrate why this was a logical and rational decision to make. It may be that the guideline is out of date or inappropriate to particular circumstances.

Evidence-based practice is the basis upon which the evidence for decision making can be demonstrated to be both rational and logical, thereby fitting in with the revised 'Bolam test' or 'Bolitho test'. It demonstrates that a healthcare practitioner has acted in accordance with the standards of their professional group.

Q How up to date do I need to be?

A There is no doubt that there is an expectation that all healthcare practitioners should be up to date in order to undertake their practice.

It would be the ideal situation if every healthcare practitioner was fully up to date; had read every article relevant to their subject; attended, or had feedback on, every seminar in their field; and was aware of every research finding appropriate to their clinical area.

Even the law knows that this standard would be impossible to achieve and does not expect you to reach this impossible standard. Given this, what standard is achievable or at least expected, for all healthcare practitioners regardless of their speciality or their area of practice?

We need to go back to the standard that is expected of all healthcare practitioners in all aspects of their practice, that of the 'Bolam test' (see **What is the legal standard I have to reach in my practice? [p. 46]**). What would a reasonable healthcare practitioner having the same skills as you and working in the same speciality consider to be appropriate and reasonable in keeping up to date? Provided that this can withstand logical scrutiny, the 'Bolitho test', then we can expect this to be accepted in a court of law, if it were challenged.

You will note that it is all about reasonableness; the reasonable practitioner considering what is reasonable to achieve. The law may be said to love reasonableness. This is because by emphasising that a healthcare practitioner's actions have to be reasonable, the standard does not have to be precisely defined and then constantly changed as practice, attitudes and expectations change over the years. Rather, the standard of doing what a reasonable healthcare practitioner would do means that the standard is effectively timeless.

The point is to act reasonably in whatever you do in your practice, including keeping up to date.

One word of caution. Although the standard for keeping up to date is the 'Bolam test' and being reasonable, if there was a change in your area of practice that was so fundamental that you should know about it, for example that a particular product was not only considered ineffective but had been proved to be harmful to patients and this was communicated widely, and you continued to use the product, it is likely that this would be considered as a breach of your duty of care to your patient.

Q Can I be sued in the execution of my duties?

A The simple answer is 'yes', you can be sued whilst executing your duties.

Being sued falls within the civil law; it means that one legal person, that is an individual or an organisation, brings a case against another.

The common reason for a civil action to be started is that the party bringing the claim (the claimant) believes that they have been wronged by the party against whom they are bringing the claim (the defendant).

This sort of legal case would fall within the area of law known as 'tort'. Depending upon which definition you use, the word 'tort' comes either from the Latin or French for twisted or wrong. Negligence is the most commonly used tort. If you were being sued in the execution of your duties, it is most likely that it would be for alleged clinical negligence.

Although it is possible for you to be sued, it is not a common occurrence, despite what you might read in the papers and hear from the television. There are countless tales and urban myths of people being sued in the execution of their duties for the most trivial of mistakes. In most cases, there is no basis for these tales or myths.

For most healthcare practitioners, a negligence claim is going to be something that happens to someone else. Even for those who do become involved in a negligence claim, it is likely that this will be as part of a team of healthcare practitioners involved in the care and treatment of an individual, rather than being sued in their own right as an individual healthcare practitioner.

The fact is that, if a healthcare practitioner acts diligently within their scope of practice, fulfilling their duty of care to their patients according to the standard of care, it is unlikely that any action against them will have a chance of succeeding.

What is clinical negligence?

Negligence is a specific form of tort, where a civil action is brought by one individual against another because they believe they have suffered harm as a result of the other's actions. Being a civil action means that the person who brings the case, the claimant, has to prove their case on the balance of probabilities. As we saw in **What is the difference between criminal and civil law? (p. 17)**, the balance of probabilities means that one side's argument is believed more than the other's.

DEFINITIONS OF NEGLIGENCE

LEGAL DEFINITION

A formal legal definition of negligence would be as follows:

> Negligence means more than heedless or careless conduct, whether in omission or commission: it properly connotes the complex concept of duty, breach, and damage thereby suffered by the person to whom the duty was owing: on all this liability depends (Lord Wright in Lochgelly Iron Company v M'Mullan [1934]: 25, a case which considered whether an employer caused the death of a miner when they failed to secure the roof in an area the miner was working).

A more useful legal definition is when the action or omission of one person leads to a loss, including an injury, for another person, with that second person having a claim in law for the loss they have suffered.

EVERYDAY DEFINITION

An everyday use of the term negligence would be when a person is careless or reckless in undertaking a task that results in some measurable harm to another person.

NEGLIGENCE IN HEALTHCARE

Negligence as a legal action first arose in 1932 in the Donoghue case, which we considered in **As a healthcare practitioner, who do I have a legal duty of care to? (p. 42)**. As well as establishing the principle of when a duty of care is owed, the case established negligence as a legal action.

The reason that this case is said to have established the modern form of negligence is because it was in this case that it was held a duty of care was deemed to exist between two parties, even if there is no contractual relationship between them, and the parties are required to take due care in their dealings with each other. The establishment of a duty between individuals and the need to act in a certain way towards each other is the basis of negligence law.

NEGLIGENCE CLAIMS

Clinical negligence is merely the name given to negligence that arises within health-care practice. As in any negligence claim, there are two stages, the liability stage and the quantum stage.

The liability stage relates to the fact that the claimant has to establish liability on the part of the defendant, that is that negligence has occurred; they have to prove four elements in their claim. These elements are:

- duty of care
- breach of that duty
- harm
- causation.

To put it another way, the claimant, who will be a patient or their representative, has to prove that the defendant, a healthcare practitioner, owed them a duty of care; that this duty was breached because the care they received was below the necessary standard; that they suffered harm; and that the harm they suffered was as a result of the low standard of care they received.

All of the above elements must be proved; if the claimant is unable to prove one of these elements, their case will fail and no negligence will be found.

From **As a healthcare practitioner, who do I have a legal duty of care to?** (p. 42), we know that healthcare practitioners have a duty of care to their patients. Therefore, in a claim in clinical negligence, it is generally not difficult for the claimant to prove that the defendant owed them a duty of care.

For a claimant to establish that the healthcare practitioner has breached their duty of care, they will have to prove that care and treatment provided by the healthcare practitioner to the patient fell below the required standard. This has been discussed in **What is the legal standard I have to reach in my practice?** (p. 46).

There are various types of harm that a claimant can claim for as a result of the negligent act of another, including:

- personal injury
- damage to their property
- monetary loss, but only as a result of one of the first two types of harm.

The fact that the patient (claimant) has shown that the healthcare practitioner (defendant) owed them a duty of care, that this duty to them was breached because the healthcare practitioner's care fell below the required standard, and the patient suffered harm is not enough to successfully bring a clinical negligence claim. Causation must also be proved; that is, that the harm suffered was directly caused by the healthcare practitioner's breach of their duty of care.

The test for proving causation is generally the 'but for' test. This test asks 'but for' the breach of duty by the healthcare practitioner, would the harm suffered by the patient have occurred? If the answer is yes, then this means another factor could have caused the harm and the patient will not be able to prove their case and will have lost their claim against the healthcare practitioner. On the other hand, if the answer is no, 'but for' the breach of duty by the healthcare practitioner the harm would not have occurred, the claimant will have proved the four elements needed, established the liability of the healthcare practitioner and won their case.

The quantum stage of a negligence case only occurs once the claimant has established the liability stage. Quantum refers to the amount of damages, the monetary award, which the defendant will have to pay to the claimant. There are various factors that are taken into account when deciding upon the damages that the claimant will receive. This includes previous cases and the damages awarded in them; however, it will be the facts of the specific case that play the major part of the calculation of damages.

GROSS NEGLIGENCE MANSLAUGHTER

This is a specific criminal offence where the harm caused to the patient by the healthcare practitioner's breach of their duty of care is so severe that the patient dies. It will be tried in the criminal courts and can also result in civil action by the patient's family.

NOTE

The vast majority of clinical negligence claims never reach court. It has been estimated that less than one in twenty are heard in court. The rest are settled out of court, with the vast majority of claims being abandoned once the healthcare practitioner has given their perspective and the health records have been checked, which highlights the importance of keeping good records (see **What constitutes good record keeping? p. 142**).

Q What is the duty of candour?

A When asked why they sue or bring a complaint against a healthcare practitioner, a considerable number of patients say that it is because they want to know what happened or for someone to apologise to them. However, if a patient sues a healthcare practitioner for negligence, if they win their case, they receive damages (see **What is clinical negligence? [p. 57]**). What they won't necessarily get is an explanation of what happened or an apology.

In an attempt to reduce the number of cases coming before the Courts and to address patient concerns by encouraging a culture of transparency, honesty and openness, the government introduced a statutory duty of candour for healthcare organisations.

The duty of candour is contained in The Health and Social Care Act 2008 (Regulated Activities) Regulations 2014. Regulation 20(1) states that, 'A health service body must act in an open and transparent way with relevant persons in relation to care and treatment provided to service users in carrying on a regulated activity'. The requirement is to inform a patient, or their representatives, when something has gone wrong, including details of the incident, what the outcome for the patient is, how things may be put right, what support will be offered to the patient and an apology.

The Care Quality Commission can investigate an organisation's approach to their duty of candour as part of its oversight of healthcare providers and could even prosecute a healthcare provider who breaches the regulations.

In addition to informing and supporting patients following adverse incidents, it is anticipated that healthcare organisations will learn from the incidents and take appropriate measures to prevent them recurring. Similar provisions have been enacted in Scotland and Wales, whilst Northern Ireland has indicated its intent to do so.

The duty of candour does not extend to individual healthcare practitioners by virtue of the legislation. However, the regulatory bodies all have statements, within their respective codes of conduct, that relate to being transparent, open and honest with patients. Additionally, healthcare employers are required to have a duty of candour policy that includes details of how to report adverse incidents and the processes that need to be followed. It is an expectation that their employees will adhere to these policies.

Therefore, although the statutory duty of candour obligation is upon an organisation, healthcare practitioners have a corresponding duty of openness and honesty to their patients.

Q Is it OK to say sorry?

A This may be an odd question to raise but there appears to be a pervasive myth that you should never apologise for something that has happened to a patient. The reasoning of those who perpetuate the myth is that, if you apologise, you will be admitting and therefore accepting liability for the event. In effect, that you are saying, 'I'm sorry that X has happened and it is my fault that it did'. However, this is not the case. Saying sorry or offering an apology does not expose you to a liability that did not previously exist.

Regulation 20 (7) of the Health and Social Care Act 2008 (Regulated Activities) Regulations 2014 defines an apology as, 'an expression of sorrow or regret in respect of a notifiable safety incident'.

The myth is so pervasive that there is even a section in an Act of Parliament that is designed to counter it. Section 2 of the Compensation Act 2006 states, 'an apology, an offer of treatment or other redress, shall not of itself amount to an admission of negligence or breach of statutory duty'.

Not only can we see that saying sorry will not expose you to liability, where none existed previously, but saying sorry is actually a requirement of the duty of candour in certain circumstances (see **What is the duty of candour?** [p. 60]).

For individual healthcare practitioners, the requirement upon them to be transparent and honest with their patients, which exists in the codes of conduct from their respective regulatory bodies, means that they should offer their patients an apology when appropriate to do so. Indeed, it can be taken as a hallmark of the highest level of practice. For the patient, saying sorry or offering an apology acknowledges that the adverse event has been recognised, that the event is regretted and that a remedy is being sought.

Q

What is vicarious liability?

A

Vicarious liability is a throwback to the days of master and servants, when a master was responsible for all the acts of his servant. In the modern form, vicarious liability means that an employer is liable for the acts of their employees, which are undertaken as part of their contractual duties. This includes acts of negligence by the employee.

There are limitations on the scope of vicarious liability. Essentially, if the act undertaken by the employee was one that was ordered or sanctioned by the employer, the action of the employee will be one that falls within the employer's vicarious liability, even if the employee undertakes it in a manner that was not authorised, as long as the employee was acting in the course of their employment at the time of the event.

If a healthcare practitioner breached their duty of care to a patient, for instance by giving the wrong drug to a patient, vicarious liability would mean that it is the employer who is liable for that act of negligence, and for any payment that is to be made to the patient and the associated legal costs. However, it would be the healthcare practitioner who has to give evidence if the case reached court.

It is important to note that an employee must be acting in the course of their employment for the employer to be vicariously liable for their actions. Thus, if a healthcare practitioner undertook a 'Good Samaritan' act outside of the work situation (see **Do I have a duty to individuals outside my clinical practice?** [p. 44]), it is highly unlikely that this would be covered by the vicarious liability of the employer.

Therefore, before assuming any change to your role and duties, it is important that this is sanctioned by your employer and you have the benefit of your employer being vicariously liable for your actions.

Why do you want your employer to be vicariously liable for your actions? Because it means that your employer will defend your actions on your behalf and pay any associated costs, including any damages, if you were found to have acted negligently.

 Do I need an indemnity arrangement?

There are organisations that exist to specifically provide healthcare practitioners with indemnity from the costs involved when being sued or having to defend a complaint against their practice.

The Shorter Oxford English Dictionary (Onions, 1984) defines 'indemnity' as, 'security or protection against contingent hurt, damage or loss'. From the health-care practitioner's perspective, indemnity does not refer to the protection of their reputation and practice, but rather to the reassurance of knowing that any financial aspect of the action against them will be met by their indemnity provider.

When you have an independent indemnity arrangement in place, you will have paid a fee to an organisation who will then indemnify you against the costs of being sued. This may include professional and legal fees associated with being sued, as well as the actual damages that you may have to pay to a claimant. Some forms of indemnity will also cover you for formal complaints made about your practice as well as complaints made against you to your regulatory body; that is, the cost of defending these types of cases.

As well as providing different types of cover, there are also different forms of indemnity cover. Some only provide cover for as long as you pay a premium, rather like insurance cover. Others will provide cover for any event that occurred in the period that you paid a fee, even if you subsequently stop the cover. It can be seen that the latter may be a preferable form of indemnity arrangement, as you are cov-ered for any event that happens even if does not come to light for some time after the event occurred, as is often the case with claims of clinical negligence, and you have stopped paying the premium for any reason, including retirement or because you have ceased practising.

An employer such as the National Health Service (NHS) provides indemnity for the actions of its employees, as it has vicarious liability for their actions; this is often referred to as 'NHS indemnity' (formerly 'Crown Indemnity'). When work-ing for other employers, it is important that you establish whether they will provide indemnity for your actions or expect you to make your own indemnity arrangements.

Many healthcare practitioners will not need to arrange their own indemnity. If you only undertake work for an employer, such as the NHS, and do not undertake anything that is outside of your contract of employment or scope of duties, or would never contemplate acting outside of your work area, it is unlikely that you would need independent indemnity protection, as cover provided by your employer will be sufficient for your practice. Indeed, many healthcare practitioners can go through the whole of their career without the need for the protection that is provided by non-employer indemnity arrangements.

However, if your employer were to criticise you, you may wish to have support to deal with the allegation. If you have to defend yourself in a regulatory body fitness to practise investigation, it is unlikely that your employer will offer assistance. You may undertake additional work, agency or voluntary, outside of your employment contract. Therefore, although the indemnity you receive from your employer is invaluable, it may not be enough for all your needs and this is where the indemnity arrangements from the various organisations that provide it come into effect.

You may find that in addition to the indemnity you have from your employer, your professional organisation also provides indemnity for you. If this is so, check what indemnity they provide you with.

As well as the support and financial aspects of indemnity arrangements that you may want, there are other reasons why you need an indemnity arrangement. Since April 2014 for the Health and Care Professions Council, August 2015 for the General Medical Council and April 2016 for the Nursing and Midwifery Council, having an indemnity arrangement in place has been a compulsory aspect of registering and remaining on the registers. The indemnity offered by the NHS fulfils the requirement for most healthcare practitioners.

Indemnity arrangements will not prevent you from being sued or having a complaint made against you, but it provides support, both in terms of having someone to support you through the process and financial support.

SUMMARY

- Healthcare practitioners have a duty of care to their patients and those who may be affected by their actions.
- There is no legal obligation to assume a duty of care outside the work situation, but the regulatory bodies require a healthcare practitioner to do so.
- To meet the legal standard of care, a healthcare practitioner must reach the standard of the ordinary competent practitioner professing to have the skills and knowledge required to undertake the specific action performed, and this standard must be capable of withstanding logical scrutiny.
- Healthcare practitioners should take reasonable steps to assist their patients but do not have to risk personal injury to care for them.
- Trainee and student healthcare practitioners are held to the same standard as their more experienced colleagues, the 'Bolam test'. However, they can meet the standard by doing what other reasonable trainees and students would do in the same circumstances.
- If you take on an advanced role or practice, the standard you have to meet does not change but the peer group you will be judged against does. You will be judged against those who normally undertake the role or practice you are undertaking.
- Where a task is delegated, the healthcare practitioner who delegated the task and the one who accepts it are both liable for their actions

- There is no concept of team liability in law and each member of a multidisciplinary team is liable for their own actions and role within that team.
- Evidence-based practice is the basis by which a healthcare practitioner can demonstrate that their practice has a logical and rational basis for meeting the standard of care.
- Healthcare practitioners need to ensure that they keep up to date with advances in their area of practice and are aware of any fundamental changes.
- Healthcare practitioners can be sued in the execution of their duties, but this is not a common occurrence.
- 'Clinical negligence' refers to when a patient sues a healthcare practitioner for harm caused by the healthcare practitioner's failure to meet the required standard of care.
- The duty of candour is a statutory obligation for a healthcare organisation to be transparent and open with patients following adverse events. A corresponding duty exists for healthcare practitioners through their respective codes of conduct.
- Saying sorry does not expose a healthcare practitioner to liability that did not previously exist.
- 'Vicarious liability' refers to situations such as when an employer is liable for the actions of their employees.
- Indemnity arrangements provide support for healthcare practitioners facing negligence claims and, in some instances, against complaints or fitness to practise investigations. Most healthcare practitioners will have an indemnity arrangement through their employer, although this may be limited to cover if sued.

REFERENCES

Bolam v Friern Hospital Management Committee [1957] 2 All ER 118.
Bolitho v City and Hackney Health Authority [1998] AC 232.
Caparo Industries PLC v Dickman and others [1990] 1 All ER 568.
Compensation Act 2006.
Donoghue v Stevenson [1932] AC 562.
F v West Berkshire Health Authority [1989] 2 All ER 545.
Hall v Brooklands Auto-Racing Club [1932] All ER 208.
Health and Care Professions Council (2016) *Standards of conduct, performance and ethics*. Health and Care Professions Council: London.
Jones v Manchester Corporation [1952] 2 QB 852.
Lochgelly Iron Company v M'Mullan [1934] AC 1.
Maynard v West Midlands Regional Health Authority [1984] 1 W.L.R. 634.
Nettleship v Weston [1971] 3 All ER 581.
Nursing and Midwifery Council (2018) *The Code*. Nursing and Midwifery Council: London.
Onions, C.T. (ed) (1984) *The Shorter Oxford English Dictionary*. Clarendon Press: Oxford.
Public Interest Disclosure Act 1998.
Social Action, Responsibility and Heroism Act 2015.
The Health and Social Care Act 2008 (Regulated Activities) Regulations 2014 (SI 2014/2936).
Wilsher v Essex Area Health Authority [1986] 3 All ER 801.

CONSENT

Consent is a fundamental ethical and legal concept within the healthcare practice. This chapter discusses the importance of consent to patients and healthcare practitioners, and how legally valid consent can be obtained from patients. It also considers the different legal positions of adults and children in relation to providing or withholding consent.

QUESTIONS COVERED IN CHAPTER 4

- Why is consent important in healthcare practice?
- What criteria must be fulfilled for consent to be legally valid?
- What is the legal definition of competence?
- How is competence assessed?
- Who can determine a patient's competence?
- How much information needs to be given to the patient?
- How do I know if the patient's consent is truly voluntary and not given under duress?
- Who should obtain consent from the patient?
- In what ways can a patient give consent?
- Can a patient refuse treatment?
- Can a patient withdraw their consent?
- Are children able to consent to their own treatment?
- Can a child refuse treatment?
- What if parents disagree on the treatment of their child?
- As a brief review, who can consent to and who can refuse treatment?
- Are there any circumstances in which someone can consent on behalf of an adult patient?
- What is a living will or advance decision?
- Do next of kin have any legal status?
- Does consent need to be obtained in an emergency?
- How can a healthcare practitioner lawfully treat an incompetent patient?

Q Why is consent important in healthcare practice?

A Consent in a healthcare context has both an ethical and a legal perspective.

From an ethical perspective, every individual has a right to determine what happens to their body so far as they are able to make that determination. This is known as 'the principle of self-determination' and is a fundamental aspect of ethics related to autonomy. It implies that the individual has the ability to make reasoned choices. Consent is the embodiment of that ethical principle.

A legal definition of consent is, 'compliance with or deliberate approval of a course of action' (Curzon, 1994). However, this is not a particularly helpful definition when you consider it in relation to the ethical principle of self-determination, as it does not indicate that the consent has to be voluntary. Indeed, under this definition, any action where one was coerced could be seen as consent to that action. It would imply that you could put another individual under pressure or influence to get them to perform a particular action and that this would be seen as them consenting to that action.

A more useful definition is that offered by the Department of Health and Welsh Office, which states that, 'consent is the voluntary and continuing permission of the patient to receive a particular treatment, based on an adequate knowledge of the purpose, nature, likely effects and risks of that treatment including the likelihood of its success and any alternatives to it. Permission given under any unfair or undue pressure is not consent' (Department of Health and Welsh Office, 1999: 67, paragraph 15.13).

This is an improvement over the legal definition of consent presented above as it states that the consent must be voluntary and continuing. It also acknowledges that once consent has been given, this is not the end of the matter as the patient must continue to give their consent to any procedure until it is complete. Additionally, the consent relates to a particular procedure; consent is not a blanket permission given to the healthcare practitioner. If an individual consents to be treated by a healthcare practitioner, that consent does not mean that the healthcare practitioner has consent from the patient to perform any procedure or treatment that they seek to provide or perform, rather consent is specific to a particular procedure and is needed for each and every procedure.

A 1914 case in the United States of America, which determined whether a surgeon can remove a tumour when the patient has not consented to its removal but is anaesthetised so that it can be examined, established the legal recognition of self-determination when Justice Cardozo stated that:

> Every human being of adult years and sound mind has a right to determine what shall be done with his own body; and a surgeon who performs an operation without his patient's consent commits an assault (Schloendorff v Society of New York Hospital, 1914: 126).

Although this case is American and was decided over one hundred years ago, it still has relevance to the modern healthcare practitioner working in the United Kingdom

(UK) as it is referred to in UK cases. If the healthcare practitioner fails to obtain consent for a procedure or treatment that they undertake on a competent patient, they can expose themselves to legal action by the patient and/or possible action by their regulatory body. As the quotation notes, performing a procedure without the patient's consent is an assault; this is a criminal act and in addition the patient may bring a civil action for negligence, trespass or battery.

In English law, an assault is when one person causes another to be fearful of physical force or violence; whereas battery is when one person commits physical force on another without their consent. Battery can exist with the slightest application of physical force, even if there is no harm caused to the other person. Both terms are often used interchangeably although, as shown, they have specific legal meanings. It is the legal meaning that will be used throughout this book.

Consent is permission from a patient for a healthcare practitioner to undertake some form of treatment on them. Consent can be seen to be important for the patient as it provides them with legal recognition for their ethical right of self-determination. For the healthcare practitioner obtaining legally valid consent, that is consent which has been obtained in the correct manner, protects them from both legal action and action by their regulatory body. Consent is part of the relationship between the patient and the healthcare practitioner; it also represents the highest level of practice.

What criteria must be fulfilled for consent to be legally valid?

As we will see throughout this book, until they are superseded, legal principles remain valid, often for a considerable amount of time. Although the following could be said to be a dated quotation, from a legal perspective, it is a seminal quotation and still valid as the principles remain unchanged.

There are four basic legal principles regarding consent within healthcare, which must be fulfilled for the permission given by the patient to be valid. These four principles are:

- The person who provides the consent must be competent to do so;
- The person consenting must be adequately informed about the nature of the procedure or treatment;
- The person must be acting voluntarily; and
- The person must not be providing their consent under duress or undue influence (Kennedy and Grubb, 1998: 111).

Although there are four principles and, from a legal perspective, the third and fourth principles listed above are entirely separate; for practical purposes, they are the same. A court would see them as separate because, legally, it would be possible to be acting voluntarily if you were under duress. For example, if someone held a family member hostage and told you to rob a bank, legally you have a choice whether to rob the bank or not. Yes, you are under duress, but you still have a choice to act or not; this choice makes your actions voluntary. It is a legal distinction that is of no practical concern to the healthcare practitioner.

If the patient is competent, has been given adequate information regarding their condition and the proposed treatment and is acting voluntarily, then the consent they provide would be legally valid.

Treatment which has been provided after legally valid consent has been given by the patient is termed 'voluntary treatment'. Without legally valid consent, the treatment would be involuntary.

What is the legal definition of competence?

There are differences in the legal competence of an individual dependent upon whether that person is an adult or a child. A later question will consider the position regarding children, but this question will concentrate on competence in adults.

CAPACITY AND COMPETENCE

From a legal standpoint, there are subtle differences between capacity and competence. For instance, the Mental Capacity Act 2005 uses the term 'capacity', whilst children are deemed to have Gillick Competence when they are able to make a decision for themselves (see **Are children able to consent to their own treatment? [p. 82]**). For ease, this book uses the term 'competence' throughout, except when included in a quotation.

In **What criteria must be fulfilled for consent to be legally valid? (p. 68)** we found that for consent to be legally valid one of the criteria that has to be fulfilled is that it is given by someone who is competent. Yet, what is competence and how do you know that the patient you are going to treat is competent to give consent?

In a day-to-day context, mental competence means the ability to make decisions or take actions affecting daily life: when to get up, what to wear, what to eat, whether to go to the doctor when feeling ill, and so on. In a legal context, it refers to a person's ability to do something, including making a decision, which may have legal consequences for the person themselves or for other people.

Until the commencement of the Mental Capacity Act 2005, which became fully in force on 1st October 2007, the law around competence to consent was based on common law principles. This means that it was based on judgments, or decisions, made in cases that came before the Courts. A leading case that provided clarity on the legal definition of competence concerned Mr C.

CASE NOTE 4.1

RE C (ADULT: REFUSAL OF MEDICAL TREATMENT) [1994]

Mr C was a 68 year old who suffered from paranoid schizophrenia and was an inpatient in a secure hospital. He developed gangrene in his right foot and was assessed by a surgeon who determined that Mr C only had a 15 per cent chance of survival if he did not have a below knee amputation. Mr C refused to have an amputation. The hospital arranged for Mr C to receive treatment with antibiotics, which avoided the immediate need for amputation, but refused to give Mr C an assurance that his leg would not be amputated as they were concerned that the gangrene would become more progressive. The hospital contended that Mr C's competence and ability to make a decision was affected by his mental illness and that he did not appreciate the seriousness of his condition or his risk of death. An application for an injunction to prevent the hospital performing an amputation was made to the court on Mr C's behalf.

The court needed to consider whether Mr C was competent or not to refuse the treatment he was being offered, or whether his competence was so affected by his mental condition and this meant that he failed to understand the information he was being given and he was unable to make a decision for himself. It was decided that Mr C's competence was affected by his paranoid schizophrenia, but not to the extent that he lacked sufficient understanding of his condition and the proposed treatment, the amputation. In fact, it was decided that he was able to understand, retain, believe and consider the information he was provided with, and was able to make a decision based on that information.

It was determined that Mr C had the competence to make a decision regarding his leg and an injunction was served preventing the hospital from amputating his leg without his written consent.

The case of Mr C resulted in what has become known as the 'Re C three-stage test of competence':

- the person must be able to comprehend and retain the relevant information
- they must believe the information they are given
- they must be able to weigh the information they have been given in the balance so as to arrive at a choice regarding the proposed treatment, balancing both risks and needs.

The 'Re C three-stage test of competence' was applied in adult cases concerning competence and in some child cases. Although the 'Re C three-stage test of competence' has been confirmed by the Court of Appeal since the original case and has been used in many cases since its introduction, the legal framework with regard to competence and the assessment of competence is now contained within the Mental Capacity Act 2005.

The first principle in the Mental Capacity Act 2005 is the fact that everyone is presumed to have competence unless, and until, it can be proved otherwise (Section 1[2]). What this means in practice is that any and every patient is deemed competent to consent to treatments and procedures, unless and until they have been declared incompetent. Some people may need help or support, such as simplified language, charts and diagrams or sign language, to be able to make a decision or communicate it, but the need for help and support does not automatically mean that they cannot make that decision.

The Mental Capacity Act 2005 does not provide a positive definition of competence, instead it defines it in the negative. By this I mean that the Mental Capacity Act 2005 does not provide a definition of what competence is but defines when a person lacks competence. That definition is, a person lacks competence, 'if at the material time he is unable to make a decision for himself in relation to the matter because of an impairment of, or a disturbance in the functioning of, the mind or brain' (Section 2[1]).

Section 2(2) of the Mental Capacity Act 2005 clarifies that it does not matter whether the, 'impairment or disturbance is permanent or temporary'. A person can lack decision-making competence even if the loss of competence is partial or temporary or if his/her competence fluctuates. In particular, it is important to realise that there are degrees of competence and it is not an all or nothing situation, a person may lack competence in relation to one matter but not in relation to others. A person who is deemed incompetent to make a decision concerning a major operation may still be competent to decide whether they wish to receive paracetamol for a headache. This is known as 'complex versus simple decision making'.

Additionally, competence can be time specific. A person may lack competence to make decisions at one point in time but hours or days later may have regained their competence. So, each decision needs to be assessed at the point in time that it needs to be made.

Legal competence therefore refers to a person's ability to be able to decide on a particular course of action based on an ability to understand, retain and believe what they are told. Along with the ability to actually arrive at a decision. Every adult is deemed to be competent unless it can be proved that they are not. Therefore, everyone over the age of 18 is able to give consent on their own behalf unless it is demonstrated that they are incompetent to do so.

How is competence assessed?

Following the introduction of the Mental Capacity Act 2005, to assess whether a patient has competence to make decisions, the following two-stage test must be used:

- Is there an impairment of, or disturbance in the functioning of, the patient's mind or brain? If so,

- Is the impairment or disturbance sufficient that the patient lacks the competence to make that particular decision?

Section 2 of the Mental Capacity Act 2005 makes it clear that a declaration of incompetence cannot be made on the basis of the patient's age, appearance, behaviour or condition alone.

THE APPLICATION OF THE TWO-STAGE TEST IS AS FOLLOWS:

STAGE ONE

First, before deciding whether a patient lacks the competence to make a decision under the Mental Capacity Act 2005, it is necessary to show that the inability to make a decision is caused by, 'an impairment of, or a disturbance in the functioning of, the mind or brain' (Section 2[1]), in other words, some form of mental disability.

This is sometimes referred to as the 'diagnostic threshold' aspect of the test. If there is no such impairment or disturbance, the patient cannot lack competence within the meaning of the Mental Capacity Act 2005.

STAGE TWO

If stage 1 of the test is met, that is the patient has some form of mental impairment or disturbance, the second stage requires it to be shown that it is the impairment or disturbance that is causing the patient to be unable to make the decision in question. Section 3 of the Act sets out the test for determining whether a patient is unable to decide for him/herself and therefore lacks competence.

This aspect of the test does not focus on the outcome or decision that the patient would make or the consequences of that decision, rather it focuses on how the patient makes their decision; as such it is often referred to as the 'functional' aspect of the test. The fact that a patient makes a decision that others would regard as being irrational or inappropriate does not in itself mean that the patient lacks competence to make that decision. In fact, patients are allowed to make any decision they like with regard to a particular treatment, so long as they are competent to do so.

Section 3(1) of the Mental Capacity Act 2005 provides that a person is unable to make a decision if s/he is unable:

(a) to understand the information relevant to the decision,

(b) to retain that information,

(c) to use or weigh that information as part of the process of making the decision, or

(d) to communicate his/her decision (whether by talking, using sign language or any other means).

You will note that this second stage of the Mental Capacity Act 2005 test for determining competence is very similar to the 'Re C test'; common law often influences legislation as can be seen here.

You must presume that a patient is competent if they do not have any form of mental impairment or disturbance; or even if they have some form of mental disability, it does not prevent them understanding, retaining or using the relevant information in making their decision, or to communicate that decision.

Who can determine a patient's competence?

Generally, the person required to assess an individual's competence to consent will be the person who wishes to take some action in connection with the person's care or treatment, or who is contemplating making a decision on the person's behalf.

For most day-to-day actions or decisions, the carer, most directly involved with the patient at the time, rather than a healthcare practitioner, will assess the patient's competence to make the decision in question. In most circumstances, it is sufficient for the person assessing competence to hold a reasonable belief that the patient lacks the necessary competence, and they would not need to undertake a formal assessment of the patient's competence.

However, reasonable belief would not necessarily be enough for those who work within healthcare. Where consent to medical treatment or examination is required, the healthcare practitioner proposing the treatment must decide whether the patient has competence to consent and, where necessary, undertake an assessment of the patient's competence. Where an assessment is undertaken, the healthcare practitioner should record the assessment process and findings in the patient's healthcare record. The notes should include the manner in which the assessment was made, the person who made the assessment and in what capacity they did so, along with the findings.

If there is any doubt about a patient's ability to consent to their own treatment, the healthcare practitioner should obtain the advice and guidance of someone qualified to determine competence.

The more serious the nature of the decision to be made, the more formal the assessment of the patient's competence may need to be. For example, a psychiatrist or psychologist may be asked for an opinion to assist with the assessment. A professional opinion may help to justify a finding in relation to competence, but the decision as to whether someone has or lacks competence must be taken by the healthcare practitioner proposing the specific treatment.

Ultimately, if a person's competence with regard to decision making is disputed, it is a question for the Courts to decide.

In legal proceedings, the burden of proof will fall on any person who asserts that the patient lacks the competence to make a decision. The person making the assertion will have to show, on the balance of probabilities, that the individual lacks competence; that it is more likely than not that the patient lacks the competence to make the decision in question.

It is important to note that the healthcare practitioner is making an assessment with regard to the competence of the patient to make a specific treatment decision, and not with regard to the patient's competence as a whole.

If you are ever in doubt regarding a patient's competence to consent, the best course of action would be to refer the matter to someone more senior.

How much information needs to be given to the patient?

For consent provided by a patient to be legally valid, the patient will have made their decision based upon the information that they needed to reach their decision. This raises the question of how much information a healthcare practitioner needs to give to a patient.

Obviously, it is not possible to state what must be told to each individual patient as this will vary according to the patient's condition and the proposed procedure. The information provided to the patient must be related to the patient's individual circumstances. However, there are some general principles that must be adhered to.

In the case of Chatterton v Gerson [1981] (which concerned a doctor who failed to explain the risk of an operation to a patient that subsequently materialised), it was held that the patient must understand in broad terms the nature and purpose of the procedure; that is, what is to be done to them, the effects that this will have upon them and the reason(s) for the proposed treatment or procedure.

Prior to the Montgomery case (see below), a healthcare practitioner would have met their legal and professional duty if they had met the 'Bolam test' (see **What is the legal standard I have to reach in my practice? [p. 46]**). Essentially, if the healthcare practitioner had provided the same information as would be provided by other reasonable healthcare practitioners in the same circumstances, this would have been sufficient for the consent given by the patient to be considered legally valid, from the information viewpoint. The latter case of Bolitho [1998] (see **What is the legal standard I have to reach in my practice? [p. 46]**) had developed the underlying legal principle so that there had to be a logical reason for the giving or withholding of each piece of information in relation to the patient's proposed procedure or treatment.

CASE NOTE 4.2

MONTGOMERY V LANARKSHIRE HEALTH BOARD [2015]

This case concerned a woman with diabetes who was at risk of delivering a higher weight baby and therefore an increased risk of shoulder dystocia occurring. This is where the head is delivered but one or both of the shoulders remains stuck in the birth canal.

Mrs Montgomery was noted to be carrying a baby of higher weight but was not warned of the possible risk of having a vaginal delivery and given the option of having an elective caesarean delivery. Shoulder dystocia did occur during the delivery and Mrs Montgomery's baby was born with severe disabilities.

The doctor who was looking after Mrs Montgomery said that she did not discuss the risk of shoulder dystocia with any of her patients because it was a small risk, and if she did, patients would opt for elective caesarean delivery and she did not believe this was in their interests. Mrs Montgomery said that if she had been aware of the risk she would have elected for a caesarean delivery.

The case was heard in the Supreme Court and they found in favour of Mrs Montgomery. This means that using the 'Bolam test', that is practising in line with what other healthcare practitioners would do, is no longer sufficient with regard to information giving. Instead, the information provided to a patient has to be specific to that individual patient according to their needs, concerns and desire for information.

The judgment in the Montgomery case only allows healthcare practitioners, 'to withhold from the patient information as to a risk if he reasonably considers that its disclosure would be seriously detrimental to the patient's health' (Montgomery v Lanarkshire Health Board [2015]: paragraph 88).

For healthcare practitioners and their patients, this means that, although not every piece of information regarding a procedure has to be given to the patient, the patient can expect to receive information that they consider they need to be able to decide whether to accept the treatment or not.

Examples of the sort of information that needs to be provided to a patient, expanding on those from Chatterton v Gerson [1981], include:

- the nature of the patient's condition that causes them to require the proposed treatment or procedure
- the nature of the procedure
- the reason for the procedure
- the benefits and risks of having the procedure against the benefits and risks of not having it
- the time element regarding the need for a decision. Is the procedure needed immediately, soon, or can the patient take their time in reaching a decision?

- the fact that the patient has a choice and if they decide not to proceed with the proposed treatment, what other treatment they could be provided with
- any common complications or side effects of the treatment, along with how these can be managed
- any future treatment they may need.

Healthcare practitioners should try not to overload the patient with information; some people find it more difficult to make a decision the more information they have. However, you need to ensure that you give patients the necessary information they need.

If the patient asks a question about their treatment, you are expected to provide them with the appropriate answer or have a sound reason for not doing so (see above). Where you do not know the answer to a question, inform the patient that you will find the answer for them and do so.

In essence, you need to discuss the proposed treatment or procedure with the patient, taking time to explain the relevant information that they need in order to be able to make their own decision.

The way in which you provide the information is also relevant. You should ensure that you provide the information to the patient in a manner in which they will understand it. This may mean presenting the information in non-verbal forms, if the patient is unable to understand verbal information. If the patient does not understand English, you may have to use an interpreter, if one is available, even by telephone or a family member to translate. There are issues with using family members as you do not know the motives of the family member. For example, the family may be waiting for your patient to die so that they can inherit and therefore do not accurately convey the patient's wishes to you in an effort to speed up this process; although we would hope this is unlikely, you cannot be sure. In addition, you could be breaching the patient's confidence. However, if you do not provide the information to the patient in a manner that they can understand, it would not be possible to state that you had provided the patient with adequate information upon which they could base their decision regarding their treatment. Therefore, their consent may be invalid and you would not have any legal basis upon which to treat them.

INFORMED CONSENT

You may have heard about informed consent. Informed consent from a legal perspective is an American concept and there is at present no principle of informed consent within English law. Whilst the Montgomery case has moved informed consent a step or two closer, it has not changed this fact, as it is still permissible to withhold information from patients in limited circumstances.

It is important to reiterate that, whilst it may be ethically or professionally responsible to utilise the principle of informed consent, there is no legal requirement or expectation to do so. Indeed, it can be argued that informed consent is unobtainable in everyday healthcare practice. This is because it is often not possible to provide the patient with *all* the information regarding a particular procedure or treatment. From an ethical perspective, it is the patient's ability to retain and understand information that ensures they are 'informed'.

When you read about 'informed consent' in government publications, regulatory body guidance or your employer's documents, they are usually referring to the principles of valid or legal consent that have been outlined above. 'Informed consent' has come to be used as shorthand for saying that the patient has the right to be involved in decisions regarding their care and treatment and that, as part of this involvement, they have the right to consent to or refuse particular treatments.

Q

How do I know if the patient's consent is truly voluntary and not given under duress?

A

As we have already seen, consent is not legally valid unless it is voluntary and given without any duress. Undue pressure or influence by the healthcare practitioner, or any other person, on the patient will render the patient's consent invalid.

In 1992 a case was heard in the Courts that had to determine if a patient was being influenced to not have a blood transfusion.

CASE NOTE 4.3

RE T (ADULT: REFUSAL OF MEDICAL TREATMENT) [1992]

T was 34 weeks pregnant when she had a car accident and was injured. Although not a Jehovah's Witness herself, she was brought up by her mother who was. After being alone with her mother, T informed a nurse that she did not want a blood transfusion. T went into labour and it was decided a caesarean section was needed. T had time alone with her mother and told the doctors that she did not want a blood transfusion. T signed a form to this effect but was not told that she might need a blood transfusion to save her life. T was admitted to intensive care after the caesarean section where she was sedated and ventilated. She needed a blood transfusion but was not given one because of her previous refusals. T's father and boyfriend made an emergency application to the court to authorise the blood transfusion. The judge authorised this in T's best interests. T subsequently appealed the decisions made on her behalf.

It was held that T's mother was influencing her to refuse to have a blood transfusion due to the mother's religious beliefs. Undue pressure or influence can be exerted to make a patient refuse a particular treatment, but it can also be used to make the patient consent to a proposed treatment. Either would render the patient's consent unlawful.

Ultimately, you may not know the reason why the patient has given their consent, and therefore cannot be sure that the patient has given their consent voluntarily without duress. Whether an individual has acted voluntarily is a matter of fact that will, if necessary, be decided by the court.

You need to assure yourself that your patient is acting voluntarily in providing their consent for any procedure. Your decision should be based on your knowledge of the patient, however slight, and all the relevant circumstances. If you believe that the patient has been subject to undue pressure, either to consent or to refuse treatment, you need to act accordingly. For instance, if you believe that the patient has been coerced into consenting then you should not perform the procedure until you have been able to assess the patient away from the source of the pressure. If you have any doubt, you should consult with another healthcare practitioner.

Although you will want to act for the benefit of the patient, you need to consider your own situation. If you perform a procedure on a patient who has refused to provide consent, even if you believe that the reason for this is undue pressure, you will be committing a possible assault and/or battery. Likewise, if you do not provide care to a patient who is requesting it of you, even where you believe this is due to undue pressure, you could be subject to an action for negligence. You therefore need to ensure that you protect yourself from possible criminal charges or a civil action. As to how you do this involves the 'Bolam test' again (see **What is the legal standard I have to reach in my practice? [p. 46]**).

The 'Bolam test' is a standard by which healthcare practitioners are judged against others who profess to have the same knowledge, skills and abilities. Essentially, if other healthcare practitioners would have reached the same conclusion regarding the voluntariness of the patient's consent as you, then you would have passed the 'Bolam test'. This means that your action would be judged to be in accordance with a responsible body of opinion and legally acceptable. For example, consulting with a colleague is likely to be considered an action which demonstrates this.

If you are working alone, the best course of action would be to contact a manager, supervisor or team centre and discuss the situation with another healthcare practitioner there, preferably someone senior where possible. This would also be an action that can be judged against the 'Bolam test'. If this was an option available to you and you did not do it, your actions could be considered unreasonable.

Who should obtain consent from the patient?

This is an easy question to answer; you, if you are going to provide the care and/or treatment.

The general principle is that the healthcare practitioner who is going to perform the procedure or treatment should be the one that obtains consent from the patient. This is because, as we saw in **How much information needs to be given to the patient? (p. 74)**, for consent to be legally valid, information about the procedure has to be provided to the patient so that they can decide whether to give or withhold their consent. If someone else obtained the consent for you, how would you know what information the patient had been given, and how would you know that the patient has received the information that you would want them to have?

However, it is acceptable practice for consent to be obtained from the patient by a healthcare practitioner who can perform the procedure, but who may not necessarily be the one who is going to perform it. The reason for the requirement that consent is obtained by someone who can perform the procedure is so that they can explain the procedure to the patient and answer any questions that the patient may have regarding the procedure. For consent to be legally valid, the adequate information requirement must be met. If the healthcare practitioner obtaining the consent is not able to explain the procedure or to answer any questions from the patient, then this requirement will not be met and the consent would not be legally valid.

Although it is legally permissible for someone else to obtain the consent from a patient for a procedure that you are going to undertake, it is your responsibility to ensure that there is a valid consent from the patient before you commence the procedure.

In what ways can a patient give consent?

There are two ways in which consent may be said to be obtained, expressly and implied. Although strictly speaking, as we will see, implied consent is not true consent from the patient.

There are two ways in which a patient may expressly provide their consent. This is either in writing or verbally. Even for a major operation, for instance open heart surgery, consent does not have to be written for it to be legally valid. Whilst your local policy may dictate that consent for all operations has to be written, and it would be inadvisable for any healthcare practitioner to disregard their local policy, there are very few instances where consent has to be written for it to be legally valid. For most circumstances, oral consent is as legally valid as if the consent had been put in writing.

As consent does not have to be put in writing to be legally valid, written consent does not mean that legally valid consent has been obtained. A signed consent form is documentary evidence that there has been a discussion, not that the patient has given legally valid consent. A form that provides evidence that a discussion was had with the patient and outlines that discussion, and the patient's decision, is a valid reason for using consent forms.

For consent to be valid, whether written or oral, the consent given must have the necessary qualities of consent about it. These qualities, described as the basic legal principles of consent, have been outlined in **What criteria must be fulfilled for consent to be legally valid? (p. 68).**

One reason for having written, as opposed to oral, consent is that of protection from claims by patients. It can take several years for civil cases to reach court.

In these circumstances, it is often difficult to rely upon one's memory and it is necessary to refer to the patient's medical notes. Having the consent form in the notes does not necessarily mean that legally valid consent was obtained, but it does suggest that there has been some dialogue between the patient and healthcare practitioner and that the patient signed the consent form for some reason. If the consent was obtained orally, it can be difficult to prove that it was in fact obtained at all, especially where it is the word of the healthcare practitioner against that of the patient. It will be a case of who is believed at the time by the court.

Implied consent, as was mentioned above, is not true consent from the patient, applies in the situation where the healthcare practitioner infers from the patient's actions or demeanour that they do not object to the procedure or treatment (see box below). It is important to note that the patient is merely not objecting to the procedure or treatment; this is vastly different from giving their permission for the procedure or treatment to be performed. Therefore, implied consent should be utilised for minor procedures or treatments only. Silence on the part of the patient should not be taken as implied consent. From a legal perspective, expressly given consent is always preferred to implied consent because it does not rely upon an inference by the healthcare practitioner as to what a patient wants, but an action by the patient to actively state that they wish to have the proposed treatment or procedure.

IMPLIED CONSENT OR NOT?

Mabel (your patient) requires her blood pressure to be taken. As you approach Mabel you inform her that you need to 'take' her blood pressure. On hearing this, she raises her arm, pushes back the sleeve of her nightdress and offers you her arm. You place the cuff around Mabel's arm and proceed to measure her blood pressure. At the end of the procedure, you help Mabel to readjust the sleeve of her nightdress.

At no time do you ask Mabel for her consent and, consequently, at no time does she expressly consent to the procedure. However, what else could you imply from Mabel's actions, other than that she did not object to you taking her blood pressure at that time? This is an example of implied consent. It would be appropriate to rely upon it with this type of procedure because there is little or no harm that could befall Mabel and it is a routine procedure that Mabel has probably permitted on numerous occasions previously.

To turn implied consent into express consent does not involve anything overly elaborate. It would be a simple matter of when approaching Mabel, instead of informing her that you need to 'take' her blood pressure, you rephrase it so that you ask her a question along the lines of, 'Mabel I need to take your blood pressure, is it okay for me to do so?'. When Mabel says 'yes that would be alright', you have her expressly given consent.

Q

Can a patient refuse treatment?

A

A patient's ethical and legal right to consent to treatment also provides them with the basis for refusing treatment. Where a competent adult patient has refused treatment, it is not possible to treat that patient.

The healthcare practitioner's ability to treat patients in their best interests is limited by the right of the patient to refuse treatment. What this means is that, if the patient is competent to consent, it is not possible to treat them in their best interests when they refuse treatment.

A key case in the development of the right to refuse treatment is that of Re T [1992], which we looked at when considering whether consent is voluntarily given. In this case Lord Donaldson stated that:

> An adult patient who ... suffers from no mental incapacity has an absolute right to choose whether to consent to medical treatment, to refuse it or to choose one rather than another of the treatments being offered. ... This right of choice is not limited to decisions which others might regard as sensible. It exists notwithstanding that the reasons for making the choice are rational, irrational, unknown or even non-existent (Re T [1992]: 652–3).

Essentially, a competent adult patient may refuse to consent for any treatment or procedure, even that which is life saving, for any reason whatsoever. It does not matter that others do not agree with or understand the patient's reasons for refusing to consent; the patient is under no obligation to explain their reasons.

The legal principle of refusal of treatment where the refusal would result in harm to the patient was considered and affirmed in the more recent case involving Ms B.

CASE NOTE 4.4

RE B (ADULT: REFUSAL OF MEDICAL TREATMENT) [2002]

Ms B was a 43 year old who had become tetraplegic as a result of a cervical spine cavernoma. As a consequence, she was transferred to an intensive care unit where she became dependent upon artificial ventilation. She had surgery to remove the cavernoma and was able to move her head and speak afterwards but remained completely paralysed from the neck down. Ms B issued formal instructions to have her artificial ventilation switched off even though she was aware that this would most likely result in her death. Despite being assessed as competent to make treatment decisions, the clinicians treating her refused to accede to her request, leading to Ms B seeking a court declaration that she was being treated unlawfully as she was competent and not consenting to the artificial ventilation.

The court held that, 'the right of a competent patient to request the cessation of treatment had to prevail over the natural desire of the medical and nursing profession to try to keep her alive'. If a competent patient has been 'given the relevant information and offered the available options, [and chooses] to refuse treatment, that decision has to be respected', even if the healthcare practitioners involved are of the belief that treatment is preferable (Re B [2002]: 450).

A patient is entitled to refuse treatment at any time; the only consideration is that they are provided with sufficient information on which to base their decision. A healthcare practitioner is entitled to advise the patient and to express their opinions, but they have to ensure that this does not stray into what may be considered to be undue influence or coercion see **How do I know if the patient's consent is truly voluntary and not given under duress? [p. 77]**).

Q

Can a patient withdraw their consent?

A

After consent has been given, for it to continue to be valid, it has to be enduring. Provided that the patient remains competent, the principle of self-determination provides them with the right to withdraw that consent, up to and including the point at which the procedure is to commence and, in some circumstances, even after treatment has commenced.

Any withdrawal of consent should be treated as if there had been no consent in the first place. To continue treatment after a patient has withdrawn their consent would be unlawful and constitute grounds for possible civil and/or criminal action against the healthcare practitioner. However, it may not always be possible to simply stop treatment after it has been started.

If the procedure has commenced and the patient signals that they are withdrawing their consent, provided that they remain competent, for instance they have not been given any medication that may affect their ability to make a decision, their withdrawal should be taken as the removal of their consent and all steps taken to end the procedure. This would not mean that the healthcare practitioner simply stops what they were doing, for instance leaving a wound half sutured and the needle still in the patient's skin! However, the minimum that is necessary to safely discontinue the procedure should be undertaken and nothing more.

Whilst it would be permissible for the healthcare practitioner to enquire as to why the patient wants the procedure to stop, and for the healthcare practitioner to explain the risks associated with stopping, they should be careful not to put the patient under duress to continue with the procedure. Remember, as stated in **How do I know if the patient's consent is truly voluntary and not given under duress? (p. 77)**, that any consent given under duress would not constitute legally valid consent.

Q

Are children able to consent to their own treatment?

The first point to note is that only competent individuals can give consent. If an individual is deemed incompetent, then they are not able to give consent for the proposed treatment or procedure regardless of their age.

Section 105 of the Children Act 1989 states that anyone under the age of 18 is a child, sometimes referred to as a 'minor'. That said, we need to consider children in two distinct groups: those aged 16–18 and those aged under 16.

CHILD AGED 16–18

Although strictly speaking anyone aged 16 to 18 is classified as a child in the eyes of the law, with regard to consent, they are deemed to have the competence to be able to give their consent for procedures and treatment for themselves, and it is not necessary to obtain consent from a parent or guardian (Family Law Reform Act 1969, Section 8).

CHILD AGED UNDER 16

There is no automatic right in law for those under the age of 16 to be able to give consent on their own behalf. In order to do so, the child under 16 has to prove that they have the competence to do so. This is the only group of individuals who have to prove their competence to consent; for everyone aged 16 and over, their competence to consent is presumed.

Competence in the under-16-year-old child is based upon the child being able to demonstrate to the healthcare practitioner that they have the intellectual and emotional maturity to make a decision regarding their own condition and treatment. The legal principle whereby children under the age of 16 can provide their own consent arises from the Gillick case.

CASE NOTE 4.5

GILLICK V WEST NORFOLK AND WISBECH AREA HEALTH AUTHORITY AND ANOTHER [1985]

Following a circular issued by the Department of Health and Social Security to Health Authorities, which stated that it was not unlawful for general practitioners to issue contraceptives to a girl under 16, Mrs Gillick sought a declaration from the court regarding the legality of the advice and whether a girl would need her parent's consent to be provided with contraception.

In the Gillick case, Lord Scarman addressed what needs to be assessed and stated that it is 'the attainment by a child of an age of sufficient discretion to enable him or her to exercise a wise choice in his or her own interests' and whether 'the child achieves a sufficient understanding and intelligence to enable him or her to understand fully what is proposed' (Gillick v West Norfolk and Wisbech Area Health Authority and another [1985]: 423).

As a result of the Gillick case, a child who is able to demonstrate that they have the necessary competence to be able to provide their own consent is often referred to as being 'Gillick competent' or having 'Gillick competence'. To be 'Gillick competent', the child would have to have the intellectual and emotional maturity to understand the nature and degree of their condition, what is being proposed regarding their treatment, including the nature and purpose of the treatment and any possible complications and side effects and the expected outcome, as well as the consequences of not having the proposed treatment. They would also have to be able to make a decision based on this information. If they are not able to arrive at a decision, they could not be deemed to be 'Gillick competent'.

The decision as to whether a particular child under the age of 16 is 'Gillick competent' is that of the healthcare practitioner who would be treating or caring for the child.

Q ### Can a child refuse treatment?

A A competent child, that is someone under the age of 18, is able to consent on their own behalf, although they are treated differently depending on whether they have reached the age of 16 or not (see **Are children able to consent to their own treatment? [p. 82]**). Those over 16 are able to consent by virtue of the Family Law Reform Act 1969, whilst those under 16 have to use the common law and be judged as being 'Gillick competent'. However, neither the statutory provision nor the common law provision mentions the child being able to withhold their consent; that is, whilst there is a legal basis for them to consent to treatment, there is no legal provision for the child to be able to refuse a treatment.

This does not mean that they cannot refuse a treatment. They can and frequently do, usually quite vocally. What it does mean is that their refusal of treatment has no legal standing as consent can be obtained from another source. As we know, for a competent adult, no-one can provide consent on their behalf. Even where the child is competent to consent and refuses, if someone with parental responsibility (see **Who is a parent and who has parental responsibility? [p. 180]**) will provide consent for the treatment, the treatment can proceed against the wishes of the child. Additionally, the Courts can provide legal authority for treatment to proceed on behalf of a child in certain circumstances.

Just because there is consent does not mean that the healthcare practitioner has to perform a procedure. A procedure can only be performed where the healthcare practitioner believes it to be in the patient's best interest *and* there is legally valid consent.

Best practice would dictate that, where a child is refusing treatment and consent is being provided by someone with parental responsibility, the healthcare practitioner must make an assessment as to whether forcing the child to have the treatment is in the child's best interests; or whether any benefit for the child of having the treatment is outweighed by the emotional trauma of being forced to have the procedure.

Where a child is deemed competent to consent, either by age or being deemed to be 'Gillick competent' and has done so, the parent cannot override the child's consent. It is only a child's refusal that may be overridden.

What if parents disagree on the treatment of their child?

Where the child is unable to consent, refuses to engage or refuses the treatment, someone with parental responsibility (see **Who is a parent and who has parental responsibility?** [p. 180]) may consent on their behalf. Parental responsibility for a single child may be held by more than one person. However, it is not legally necessary for those with parental responsibility to consult on any decision and parental responsibility may be exercised by anyone who holds it on behalf of the child.

This position was confirmed in a case involving treatment for a child, R.

CASE NOTE 4.6

RE R (A MINOR) (WARDSHIP: MEDICAL TREATMENT) [1991]

A 15-year-old girl was admitted to an adolescent psychiatric unit after attacking her father with a hammer. With her consent, she was occasionally sedated to prevent her having psychotic episodes. A decision was made that she needed to be treated with antipsychotic drugs. However, R refused these when she was in a lucid state and, because of her refusal, the hospital would not administer the drugs to her. An application was made to the court as to whether it was lawful for the drugs to be administered against R's refusal and whether a 'Gillick competent' child (see **Are children able to consent to their own treatment?** [p. 82]) could refuse treatment.

The case was heard in the Court of Appeal and, in the judgment, Lord Donaldson said that a 'Gillick competent' child had no right to refuse treatment. He stated that consent 'is merely a key which unlocks a door. ... In the ordinary family unit where a young child is the patient there will be two key holders, namely the parents, with a several as well as a joint right to turn the key and unlock the door. If the parents disagree, one consenting and the other refusing, the doctor will be presented with a professional and ethical, but not with a legal, problem because, if he has the consent of one authorised person, treatment will not without more constitute a trespass or a criminal assault' (Re R [a minor] [wardship: medical treatment] [1991]: 184).

Thus, where the healthcare practitioner has received a key from anyone with parental responsibility, or the patient themselves, they may lawfully treat the patient and do not need consent from all concerned. This does not apply where the treatment in question is non-therapeutic, for instance religious circumcision (Children Act 1989: Section 2.7). In these situations, consent is required from both parents and, if one was not willing to provide their consent, the procedure would not be able to proceed legally.

It is always good practice to discuss proposed treatment with both parents and obtain their consent; however, where there is disagreement between the parents, provided that it is a therapeutic treatment and consent can be obtained from one of the parents, it would be legally possible to proceed.

The best interests of the child should always be paramount and, although you may have consent from one parent to proceed, this does not mean that you have to; although, where you consider it in the child's best interests, that single consent will give you the legal basis to proceed with the treatment.

 Q As a brief review, who can consent to and who can refuse treatment?

A The following patients would be able to consent on their own behalf:

- competent adults
- competent children over 16 (by virtue of the Family Law Reform Act 1969)
- children under 16, but only if they have been deemed to be 'Gillick competent'.

The following can refuse to consent to treatment:

- competent adults.

The following can refuse to consent, but their refusal can be overridden by someone with parental responsibility:

- children over 16
- children under 16.

Where someone is under 18, the Courts may authorise treatment in their best interests.

 Q Are there any circumstances in which someone can consent on behalf of an adult patient?

 A If an adult patient is incompetent, in certain circumstances, it is possible for some-one else to provide consent to healthcare treatment. However, this is a very specific set of circumstances and the general principle in English law is that no-one can provide consent on behalf of another adult, competent or incompetent. This was confirmed in a case concerning Ms T.

CASE NOTE 4.7

T V T AND ANOTHER [1988]

T was a 19-year-old severely mentally handicapped woman who was unable to live independently and was cared for by her mother. When T became pregnant, because she was incompetent and unable to consent to an abortion, her mother requested that the court provide consent for the procedure.

It was held that no-one can give consent on behalf of an adult, not even the court. However, the abortion could be performed in T's best interests.

The circumstances where an individual is able to provide consent on behalf of another adult, who is incompetent, is when the incompetent person had made a 'Lasting Power of Attorney' (LPA) when they were competent. LPAs were introduced by the Mental Capacity Act 2005 and are a legal document that allows one person (the donor) to give authority to another person (the attorney) to act on their behalf. The authority can be in relation to financial affairs and/or to the welfare and healthcare of the donor; the document must explicitly state which authority is being given to the attorney.

In order to be legally valid, LPAs have to fulfil specific criteria such as: being completed on a prescribed form; by an adult; include a certificate from a third party, that is not the donor or attorney, that states the donor understands the authority they are making and is not doing so under duress; and be registered with the Court of Protection.

The effect of a valid LPA is that, once the donor becomes incompetent, any decision made on their behalf by the attorney has the same effect as if it was made by the donor themselves. This includes decisions relating to healthcare treatment; the attorney is giving or withholding consent as if they were the donor.

LPAs do not give the attorney the right to seek unlawful treatment for the donor, nor to insist upon a specific treatment that the healthcare practitioner does not believe is appropriate for the patient.

The attorney cannot use their authority if the donor is competent to make their own treatment decisions, nor can they use their authority with regard to life-sustaining treatment unless this is specifically stated in the LPA document.

An LPA, if made after an advance decision (see **What is a living will or advance decision?** [p. 88]), would render the advance decision invalid unless the option for the attorney to give or refuse consent to life-sustaining treatment is not included in the LPA.

For healthcare practitioners, if an incompetent patient has a valid LPA when considering treatment options, they must consult with the attorney and seek their consent to any proposed treatment that falls within the authority of the LPA. They should consider the attorney as if they were the patient. The attorney must always act in the best interests of the donor. If the healthcare practitioner believes that the attorney is not doing so, they can apply to the court for a declaration as to the treatment the donor requires. Whilst the court is considering its decision, the healthcare practitioner may provide the treatment that they consider is in the patient's best interests, including life-sustaining treatment.

Q What is a living will or advance decision?

A There are several terms that you may have come across that relate to broadly similar legal principles. These include advance directive, advance decision, advance refusal, advance statement and living will.

An 'advance directive' is a common law principle, whereas an 'advance decision' is the same legal principle but refers to the fact that the principle has been provided for by statute, specifically the Mental Capacity Act 2005. A 'living will' is the term used by members of the public for either an advance directive or advance decision. 'Advance refusal' is sometimes used for any or all of these. The terms refer to the same legal principle, that a competent adult is entitled to refuse treatment that is offered to them and the decision is the expression of the treatment the patient does not wish to receive. Throughout the rest of this question, the term 'advance decision' will be used.

An 'advance statement', however, is a different legal principle. An advance statement is the expression of the patient's wishes and desires; what they would like to happen to them at a time when they are unable to play an active part in their own care and treatment. It is a statement made in anticipation of the patient losing their competence to make decisions. It sets out to healthcare practitioners what the patient would like to happen in given situations.

ADVANCE DECISIONS

There is no obligation upon anyone to make an advance decision; however, a competent adult has the legal right to make one should they wish. They can be made in any way that the individual wishes as there is no prescribed form that they have to take; they can be expressed in lay terms. Unless they specifically deal with life-sustaining treatment, they do not even have to be in writing.

If the advance decision is made orally to a healthcare practitioner, a note should be included in the patient's healthcare record as to the existence and extent of the advance decision. Best practice would suggest that this is witnessed by another healthcare practitioner whenever possible.

An advance decision is a decision that is made whilst the patient is competent with regard to their future treatment and care. It should list the circumstances in which the individual would not want specific treatment or treatments, for instance if they have condition X they would not want treatment Y. Both the circumstances in which they would not want the treatment and the specific treatments being refused have to be expressly included for the advance decision to be valid.

An advance decision can be withdrawn, partially withdrawn, or altered at any time whilst the individual who made it is still competent to do so. This can be done orally or in writing, again there is no prescribed form in which this has to be done.

The advance decision does not have any legal meaning until the person loses their competence to make a decision regarding the condition and treatment that is specified in the advance decision. Provided that the advance decision is valid, and applicable to the circumstances of the patient, any refusal of treatment that has been made must be treated the same as if the patient were competent and making the refusal themselves at that time. This is because a valid advance decision is the same as the patient making a contemporaneous decision themselves and takes precedence over treating them in their best interests.

Advance decisions cannot be used when the patient still has the competence to make a decision regarding the treatment that is specified in the advance decision; or where the treatment being proposed is not specifically mentioned in the advance decision; or where the circumstances in the advance decision are not met, for example the advance decision states that it should only be in force if the patient has a specific condition which they do not have; or where there is a reasonably held belief that the patient did not contemplate the circumstances in which they are now in.

An advance decision can include refusal of life-sustaining treatments but to be legally valid this would have to be in writing and signed by the individual and witnessed, and include a statement that the individual specifically wanted to refuse the treatment even if their life was at risk.

If there is any doubt as to the validity of an advance decision, an application can be made to the Courts for a ruling. Whilst this is being decided, the healthcare team can legally undertake any treatment that they believe is in the patient's best interests, including life-sustaining treatment, even those that are specifically prohibited by the advance decision.

ADVANCE STATEMENTS

It is an established legal principle that no-one is able to demand a particular healthcare treatment; treatment is only offered by a healthcare practitioner when they believe that it will confer a benefit for the patient. A healthcare practitioner is not obliged to offer a patient a treatment that they consider to be clinically unnecessary just because the patient requests it. Therefore, an advance statement cannot be used to request a specific treatment and has no legal weight in terms of compelling the healthcare practitioner to follow all the details it includes.

However, it is a useful document for healthcare practitioners in their clinical interaction with patients as it indicates the patient's preferences, wishes and beliefs when the patient is no longer able to make decisions for themselves and can be used to determine a patient's best interests.

Q **Do next of kin have any legal status?**

A 'Next of kin' is a term that will be familiar to any healthcare practitioner and one that is recognised by members of the public. However, whilst we may all know what we are talking about when we use the term, it is not one that has a legal definition or any legal status.

When we ask a patient who their next of kin is, we generally mean who do they want to nominate as the point of contact for healthcare practitioners should the need arise.

It is not a 'title' that carries any legal standing. It certainly does not give the person nominated as the next of kin any legal right to be involved in the patient's care and treatment. In fact, it gives no legal rights to the person at all. As confirmed in the F v West Berkshire Health Authority [1989] case (see **Do I have a duty to individuals outside my clinical practice? [p. 44]**), no-one, including the Courts, can consent on behalf of an adult.

If a relative or next of kin wants to exercise any legal rights in relation to the patient's care and treatment, they need to be registered as the patient's representative via a Lasting Power of Attorney.

The only other time that a relative has any role, apart from parents as we have already seen, is in relation to patients subject to the Mental Health Act 1983 if they are the 'nearest relative' (see **Do relatives have a role in mental health care and treatment? [p. 195]**) or if they meet the criteria to be considered in a 'qualifying relationship' within the definition of the Human Tissue Act 2004 in relation to organ donation (see **How is consent obtained for the use of a patient's organs for transplant? [p. 224]**). Apart from these two specific roles for relatives, they have no legal role or rights in healthcare practice.

In summary, next of kin or relatives have no legal power over the treatment a healthcare practitioner provides to a patient; they have no legal right either to consent or to refuse to consent for those over the age of 18; and, from a legal perspective, their wishes or directions do not have to be followed.

Q **Does consent need to be obtained in an emergency?**

A If the patient is competent, yes. The fact that the situation is an emergency does not change any of the legal principles discussed previously in this chapter. If the patient is competent, that means they are able to provide consent, or to refuse treatment, and so you must obtain the patient's consent before treating them. Obviously, an unconscious patient is incompetent and different principles apply in this situation (see the next question, **How can a healthcare practitioner lawfully treat an incompetent patient? [p. 91]**).

How can a healthcare practitioner lawfully treat an incompetent patient?

It is an absolute principle of English law that once an individual has reached the age of 18 no-one can consent on their behalf, unless the person has expressly given them the right to do so by creating a Lasting Power of Attorney (see **Are there any circumstances in which someone can consent on behalf of an adult patient? [p. 86]**).

When considering the treatment of incompetent patients, we need to remember that unconscious patients are seen as incompetent in law as they would fail the Mental Capacity Act 2005 criteria described in **How is competence assessed? (p. 71)**.

Two points need to be made with regard to the treatment of incompetent patients. Firstly, it is not possible to go to the Courts and ask them for consent to treat a patient. Not even the Courts can give consent once the patient has reached the age of 18, although they are able to rule that a particular treatment would not be unlawful. Secondly, if a valid LPA is in force, consent can be obtained from the attorney. This would provide the legal basis for treating an incompetent patient.

The rest of this answer will consider situations where there is no LPA in force.

In an emergency, not only may the healthcare practitioner act but, unless there is information to the contrary, the healthcare practitioner is under a legal duty to treat patients who are incompetent to consent. Information to the contrary may be where there is an advance decision that covers the present situation or where the patient has, whilst competent, refused consent for the proposed procedure or treatment.

The legal basis on which an incompetent patient may be treated is the same whether it is an emergency situation or not. It is the common law principle of necessity, established in F v West Berkshire Health Authority [1989] (see **Do I have a duty to individuals outside my clinical practice? [p. 44]**) that gives a healthcare practitioner the legal authority to act. The healthcare practitioner may perform what is necessary, 'to preserve the life, health or well-being' of the patient (per Lord Goff in F v West Berkshire Health Authority [1989]: 565). The treatment that is performed must be in the patient's best interests. For Lord Brandon, 'the operation or other treatment will be in their [the patient's] best interests if, but only if, it is carried out in order to either save their lives, or to ensure improvement or prevent deterioration in their physical or mental health' (F v West Berkshire Health Authority [1989]: 551).

The concept of 'best interests' was further developed in relation to the treatment of MB.

CASE NOTE 4.8

RE MB [1997]

MB was a 23-year-old woman who was 40 weeks pregnant and was advised to have a caesarean section. However, because she was needle phobic, she refused the caesarean section to avoid the anaesthetic. The hospital was convinced that a caesarean section was necessary and so sought a declaration that it would be lawful to perform it.

It was held that she should be treated as incompetent due to her needle phobia and underwent the caesarean section. The court declared that best interests may be anything that preserves the life, health or wellbeing of the patient and does not necessarily have to confer a medical benefit on the patient; the benefit may also be psychological or social.

In addition to the case law above, the principle of best interests has been established in the Mental Capacity Act 2005.

We know that, where possible, the patient should be involved in decisions about their treatment. Where a patient is incapacitated but is expected to regain competence, and it is not an emergency situation, it may be thought to be best practice to wait for the patient to regain their competence before proceeding with any treatment. In most instances, this will be the case. However, Lord Goff is of the opinion that, 'where the need to care for him [the patient] is obvious … the doctor must then act in the best interests of his patient … were this not so, much useful treatment and care could, in theory at least, be denied to the unfortunate' (F v West Berkshire Health Authority [1989]: 567). However, the healthcare practitioner should do no more than is reasonably required in the best interests of the patient.

As to what a patient's best interests may be, we have to consider the actual circumstances of the patient. It is the best interests of the patient that are paramount, not whether there would be a benefit to another individual or to the healthcare practitioner or the healthcare team.

To determine a patient's best interests, consideration needs to be given to the full range of the patient's welfare and not merely the medical aspects. It is also important to reflect on all the factors that the patient would consider important and not just those that the healthcare practitioner considers important. It should take into account the patient's ascertainable wishes, values, beliefs and feelings; any physical, emotional and educational needs of the patient; the likely effect the proposed treatment or procedure may have upon the patient; the patient's age, sex, background and other appropriate characteristics; the patient's condition and the possible harm that the patient is suffering or is at risk of suffering if the proposed treatment or procedure is not undertaken; whether the patient will regain competence and if so when; and, how easy it will be to care for the patient, having had the proposed treatment or procedure or if they do not have the proposed treatment or procedure. Additionally, where appropriate, the healthcare practitioner should consult any attorney appointed under an LPA or anyone who is or has been caring for the patient, as to the wishes of the patient and what the patient's best interests may be.

The patient's best interests cannot be met by providing treatment if an advance decision exists that covers the proposed treatment or, when competent, the patient previously refused to consent to this treatment.

In summary, where the patient is incompetent, treatment can be provided to them on the basis of the principle of necessity and related to their best interests.

SUMMARY

- Consent is permission from a patient for a healthcare practitioner to provide them with treatment or a procedure.
- Consent is important from both a legal and ethical perspective and is a vital issue for any healthcare practitioner.
- For consent to be legally valid, it has to fulfil certain criteria.
- Competence refers to a person being able to decide on a particular course of action based on an ability to understand, retain and believe what they are told, along with the ability to arrive at a decision.
- Every adult is deemed to be competent unless it can be proved that they are not.
- Competence is assessed using a two-stage test, which seeks to determine if a patient has any form of mental impairment or disturbance that prevents them understanding, retaining or using relevant information to make a decision, or to communicate that decision.
- An assessment of a patient's competence to consent to a specific treatment is usually undertaken by the healthcare practitioner wishing to undertake that treatment.
- Patients should receive information relating to treatment or procedures according to what they consider they need to be able to reach a decision.
- Consent must be given voluntarily and without undue influence. A patient may be coerced into refusing or accepting treatment. Both could render any consent unlawful.
- In general, the healthcare practitioner who is proposing the treatment or procedure for the patient should discuss it with the patient and obtain their consent; if this is not possible, it should be obtained by a healthcare practitioner who is able to undertake the procedure.
- A competent patient can refuse treatment even if doing so would result in their death.
- A competent patient may withdraw their consent at any time.
- Those children who are 16 or over can consent automatically by virtue of the provisions in the Family Law Reform Act 1969. For those under the age of 16, there is an additional hurdle before they are able to consent on their own behalf;

they have to prove to the healthcare practitioner that they have the necessary emotional and intellectual maturity, known as being 'Gillick competent'.

- Whilst a child can refuse treatment, their refusal has no legal weight if someone with parental responsibility provides consent on their behalf.
- For therapeutic treatments, only one person with parental responsibility needs to provide consent for a child to be treated.
- Lasting Powers of Attorney are the only mechanism by which someone may consent on behalf of another adult.
- Advance decisions and advance statements are legal methods by which a patient may respectively refuse treatments or express their treatment wishes in anticipation of becoming incompetent in the future.
- Next of kin are not legally defined and have no legal status in relation to patients.
- Even in an emergency, consent needs to be obtained before treating competent patients.
- Where the patient is incompetent, treatment can be provided to them on the basis of the principle of necessity and related to the patient's best interests.

REFERENCES

Bolam v Friern Hospital Management Committee [1957] 2 All ER 118.
Bolitho v City and Hackney Health Authority [1998] AC 232.
Chatterton v Gerson [1981] QB 432.
Children Act 1989.
Curzon, L.B. (1994) *Dictionary of Law* (4th edition). Pitman Publishing: London.
Department of Health and Welsh Office (1999) *Mental Health Act 1983 Code of Practice.* The Stationery Office: London.
F v West Berkshire Health Authority [1989] 2 All ER 545.
Family Law Reform Act 1969.
Gillick v West Norfolk and Wisbech Area Health Authority and another [1985] 3 All ER 402.
Human Tissue Act 2004.
Kennedy, I. and Grubb, A. (eds) (1998) *Principles of Medical Law.* Oxford University Press: Oxford.
Mental Capacity Act 2005.
Mental Health Act 1983.
Montgomery v Lanarkshire Health Board [2015] UKSC 11.
Re B (adult: refusal of medical treatment) [2002] 2 All ER 449.
Re C (adult: refusal of medical treatment) [1994] 1 All ER 819.
Re MB [1997] 38 BMLR 175.
Re R (a minor) (wardship: medical treatment) [1991] 4 All ER 177.
Re T (adult: refusal of medical treatment) [1992] 4 All ER 649.
Schloendorff v Society of New York Hospital (1914) 211 NY 125.
T v T and another [1988] 1 All ER 613.

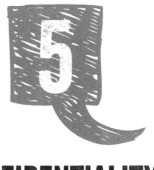

CONFIDENTIALITY

Chapter 5 is concerned with personal information that healthcare practitioners come across in the execution of their duties. It includes how they must handle confidential information, what they can legally and ethically do with confidential information, and when they are legally obliged to pass confidential information on to a third party.

QUESTIONS COVERED IN CHAPTER 5

- What is clinical confidentiality?
- Why, as a healthcare practitioner, do I need to know about clinical confidentiality?
- When does the duty of confidentiality arise?
- What are the principles of clinical confidentiality?
- What kinds of information might have the 'necessary quality of confidence' or be considered as confidential?
- What 'circumstances impart an obligation of confidence'?
- What does 'the information must have been divulged to a third person without the permission, and to the detriment, of the person originally communicating it' mean?
- What does 'the information must not be in the public domain already' mean?
- Why must it 'be in the public interest to protect the information'?
- How can information be shared without breaching confidentiality?
- Is it OK to share information that has been anonymised?
- Are there occasions when a healthcare practitioner is obliged to disclose confidential patient information?
- What is a duty to warn?
- Where there is a duty to warn, who should be told?
- What can be disclosed when fulfilling a duty to warn?
- If a patient is concerned about their confidentiality being breached, what remedies are available to them?
- What are Caldicott Guardians and how do they relate to confidentiality?
- As a healthcare practitioner, do I need to know about the Data Protection Act 2018?

(Continued)

- Do any of the principles of confidentiality change if my patient is under 18?
- Do any of the principles of confidentiality change after the death of the patient?
- Does research in the healthcare setting raise any special issues in relation to confidentiality?
- Does my duty of confidentiality to my patients end when I move employers or when I cease being a healthcare practitioner?
- As a brief review, what are the reasons or ways in which confidential information may be shared with third parties?

What is clinical confidentiality?

If something is confidential, it has an air of mystery to it. Why is it confidential? Why can't I know about it? The essence of information being confidential is that it is not shared to a wide audience but rather knowledge of it is restricted to only those who need to know. When it is divulged to another, it is done so in confidence and the secret will be kept by that person. Maintaining a confidence means not to pass on the information to which the confidence relates. The confidential information does not have to be a very big secret, just a piece of information that someone does not want to be made widely available, and therefore wants to restrict who is aware of it.

'Confidentiality' refers to the keeping of a confidence: a piece of communication between individuals that is not to be divulged to those outside of the sphere of confidence.

'Clinical confidentiality' merely refers to confidentiality in a healthcare setting. It refers to the relationship between a healthcare practitioner and a patient, the information that the former gains about the latter and what the healthcare practitioner can and cannot do with that information.

Clinical confidentiality is not a novel concept. It is a fundamental element of healthcare practice and is enshrined in the codes of conduct issued to registrants by the healthcare regulatory bodies. Indeed, it has been around since at least the fifth to third century BC as it is a principle in what could be termed the original code of conduct for healthcare practitioners, the Hippocratic Oath, which mentions keeping information obtained during the course of one's profession secret.

Given that it is such an old and established part of healthcare practice, it may be surprising to learn that in the United Kingdom there is no single piece of legislation that covers the healthcare practitioner's obligation to maintain their patient's confidentiality.

However, nothing is as simple as it first seems when considering law and ethics in healthcare. The healthcare practitioner's duty to maintain their patient's confidentiality is based in common law and the codes of conduct issued by the regulatory bodies. As we will see in the questions that follow, there are several pieces of legislation which have provisions that cover elements of the healthcare practitioner's duty to maintain patient confidentiality.

Q Why, as a healthcare practitioner, do I need to know about clinical confidentiality?

A Clinical confidentiality is an example of an ethical principle that can be said to be both deontological and utilitarian in outlook.

As a healthcare practitioner, you are expected to practise lawfully and ethically according to any additional requirements stipulated by your regulatory body. Codes of conduct require that you protect the confidentiality of your patients; you need to know what it is you are protecting and why. It is also highly likely that any contract of employment or university and student agreement will have a confidentiality clause regarding patient information gained during the course of your employment or studies built into them. If you were to breach your duty to maintain patient confidentiality, you could in theory be subject to legal, employer, university and/or regulatory body disciplinary action against you.

Additionally, as we will shortly see, there are other compelling reasons why you need to protect patient confidentiality.

We have seen earlier when discussing the question '**What are the main ethical principles relevant to healthcare practice?**' (**p. 12**) that patient autonomy is a key ethical principle in healthcare practice. Patient autonomy is concerned with patients making their own decisions relating to their healthcare. Maintaining patient autonomy is a fundamental principle of healthcare practice. Therefore, if a patient wishes the information they provide to a healthcare practitioner to remain confidential then the patient's autonomy should be respected, unless there are compelling reasons for not doing so.

Autonomy is an individual right; it pertains to a particular individual and is for their benefit. There is also a public interest or wider principle at stake in maintaining clinical confidentiality. This is based on the rationale of why patients share information with healthcare practitioners and why a healthcare practitioner needs information from a patient.

If we take the last point first, you need certain information from a patient to be able to effectively treat them. Without patient supplied information, your job would be much harder, if not impossible. How do you know what condition the patient needs treatment for if you have no information from the patient? Can you provide a certain treatment or medication if you don't know the patient's allergies or current medication?

The patient shares information with their healthcare practitioner for the same reason; they want to receive safe and effective treatment, and they know that providing certain information will assist that. However, patients provide information in the knowledge and expectation that it will only be used for their benefit and will not be shared unnecessarily or with just anyone. This includes relatives of an adult patient, the police, friends of the patient, work colleagues, in fact anyone who is not directly involved with the patient's care and treatment and in need of the information. If they did not believe this, they might be less disposed to provide you with the information that you are asking for. This would have consequences for them in that they may not want to seek treatment at all, or they may seek treatment but be less than forthcoming when asked to provide information. Either situation could result in them not receiving the treatment they need in a timely manner.

There is also a greater impact of individuals not sharing personal information to their healthcare practitioner than just the impact on their own health. This is the impact on public health. If enough individuals do not seek advice or treatment for their illnesses, because they are fearful of what will happen to their personal information, the health of the wider public may suffer as a consequence. The utilitarian argument would be that maintaining clinical confidentiality for individual patients has a positive effect for the wider public.

To provide optimum healthcare to your patients you need to maintain clinical confidentiality and, in so doing, will be protecting not only the patient in front of you but also the wider public. To maintain clinical confidentiality effectively you need to know what it is, what it covers and when it can be overridden.

Q When does the duty of confidentiality arise?

A A duty of confidentiality can arise as part of a contract. In a contract of employment, there may be a clause that requires the employee to keep information acquired during the course of their employment confidential. As an example, a nanny employed by a famous family who witnesses arguments between the parents of the child they are caring for could be restricted from passing on that information to others, including the press, by a confidentiality clause in their contract of employment. Most healthcare practitioners can expect to have a confidentiality clause in their contract of employment.

Healthcare practitioners will also have a duty of confidentiality to their patients arising from other sources. These include a confidentiality principle in the codes of conduct issued by the healthcare regulatory bodies. All the healthcare regulatory bodies have a principle relating to confidentiality that is usually along the lines of: you (as a registrant) must respect the confidentiality of patients, clients or service users. If the healthcare practitioner is working in the National Health Service (NHS), they will also be bound by the policy *Confidentiality: NHS Code of Practice* (Department of Health, 2003).

Although there is no single Act of Parliament that covers all the legal principles regarding confidentiality, there is legislation that places an obligation on individuals and organisations with regard to the confidentiality of information that they have and what they may, may not and/or have to do with that information. These include the National Health Service Act 2006, Health and Social Care Act 2012, Human Rights Act 1998, and Data Protection Act 2018.

Finally, the source of the legal obligation to keep certain information confidential (the legal duty of confidentiality) arises in the common law where it is based upon a need to protect the public interest. In respect of clinical confidentiality, the common law duty could be the most relevant as it is what would be used to demonstrate a breach of confidence; along with the duty imposed by codes of conduct for healthcare practitioners.

 What are the principles of clinical confidentiality?

Because we lack a single Act of Parliament that provides all the legal provisions that are needed to provide for a law on confidentiality, such as what legal principles apply in what circumstances, we lack the statutory guidelines that would come with such an Act. Rather, we have to turn to the common law and see how the Courts have approached the legal concept of confidentiality and how various principles have originated and developed through cases about breach of confidentiality.

This turns the way we approach the principles that underpin clinical confidentiality on its head. Rather than being able to say, 'these are the principles that you need to adhere to maintain clinical confidentiality', which is what we could expect if there was a single statutory provision for confidentiality, we have to approach it from a different angle and ask, 'What does the common law require us to prove if we were to bring a case before the court alleging that a breach of confidentiality had taken place?'.

Taking the judgments from two key cases – Coco v Clark [1968], where a breach of confidentiality was alleged in relation to engine designs, and Attorney-General v Guardian Newspapers (No. 2) [1990], which considered whether a former MI5 agent could publish his memoirs – that established the legal obligation to maintain confidentiality, five common law principles can be formulated. To establish that a duty to maintain confidentiality has been breached, and win their case, the defendant would have to prove that:

- the information has the necessary quality of confidence
- the information was imparted in circumstances importing an obligation of confidence
- they have suffered detriment because the information was divulged to a third person without their permission
- the information must not be in the public domain already
- the public interest is served by protecting the information (Cornock and Nichols, 2008).

In the questions that follow, we will explore what these five common law principles mean in the healthcare context.

 What kinds of information might have the 'necessary quality of confidence' or be considered as confidential?

 Another way of asking this question would be: What is confidential information? Unfortunately, it is not possible to point to any guidelines or a legal case or piece of legislation, and say, because of this document, we can categorically state that these types of information are considered confidential. It would be great if we could. Rather, confidential information can take a variety of forms and, in many cases, it is the context of the sharing of the information which results in it being considered confidential or not.

For instance, the Courts have declared that various types of information can be confidential.

CASE NOTE 5.1

STEPHENS V AVERY [1998]

Mrs Stephens was a close friend with Mrs Avery and, during the course of their friendship, Mrs Stephens and Mrs Avery discussed personal and intimate details of Mrs Stephens' sexual relationships, including the fact that she had had a lesbian relationship with a woman who was subsequently killed by her husband. Mrs Avery passed on this information to a national newspaper who published it. Mrs Stephens brought an action for damages against Mrs Avery, the newspaper and the newspaper editor (the defendants). The defendants' argument was that Mrs Stephens' behaviour was immoral and that, because the relationship she had with the woman was outside of her marriage, it was not protected by the law on confidential information, and that any discussion of this behaviour should be considered as gossip and therefore not protected.

The court held that personal and intimate information, in this case information about sexual conduct and sexual relationships, could be information that is confidential.

It is reasonable to regard information regarding someone's sexual conduct as being confidential to them. They should be able to choose who that personal and intimate information is shared with. In many areas of clinical practice, healthcare practitioners will find that they become privy to information of a personal and intimate nature, disclosed to them by their patients. The judgment in the Stephens case shows that this type of information has the necessary quality of confidence about it.

Notwithstanding the judgment in the Stephens case, for many years it can be said that there was a distinction between information that was held to have a quality of confidence about it, and so was protected, and private information that wasn't.

CASE NOTE 5.2

CAMPBELL V MGN LIMITED [2004]

Naomi Campbell, in the words of the judgment, 'a celebrated fashion model', brought an action against *The Mirror* newspaper for publishing photographs of her said to be leaving a Narcotics Anonymous meeting in an article that discussed her addiction and treatment. The newspaper argued that this was justified because Ms Campbell had denied that she had an addiction problem, this was evidence to the contrary and it was in the public interest to publish it. Ms Campbell argued that this was private information and sought damages.

The case was ultimately heard in the House of Lords and Ms Campbell received damages. What is of note is that, as a result of the judgment in this case, a duty of confidence can be said to extend to private information, that is information about a person's private life.

In practical terms, what this means is that almost any piece of information can be confidential, subject to exclusions that we will discuss in the questions that follow. As a healthcare practitioner, any information that you obtain as a result of your practice should be considered to have necessary quality of confidence. As such, you should not disclose any patient information to anyone else without the necessary authority to do so. We will discuss the ways in which information can legally and ethically be shared in a later question.

Q What 'circumstances impart an obligation of confidence'?

A As with the previous question, there is no single document we can inspect which will tell us all circumstances that information can be shared which impart an obligation of confidence and those circumstances which don't.

As we saw when considering if information has the necessary quality of confidence about it, there isn't a specific form of information that is automatically considered confidential. In many cases, it is the interplay of various factors that determine if information is confidential or not, and one of these factors is the way in which the information was shared or imparted to another. That said, there are some general points that can be made.

We saw in the Stephens v Avery [1998] case (see **What kinds of information might have the 'necessary quality of confidence' or be considered as confidential? [p. 99]**) that personal and intimate information can be considered confidential. Let's now see how the circumstances in which the information is shared can determine whether it should remain confidential or not.

Suppose you have a friend who has a sexually transmitted disease that you are unaware of. Your friend knows you are a healthcare practitioner and decides to tell you about their sexually transmitted disease. Would this impose a duty of confidentiality on you?

A reasonable person, and I'm not saying you are not a reasonable person, would most likely consider that this is a private conversation between two individuals and one that has the necessary quality of confidence about it. The reasonable person would not expect you to share this information with others without the consent of your friend.

Now imagine that your friend decides to tell you about the sexually transmitted disease whilst you are both in the city centre and using a loudhailer; I'm not sure why they would do this but let's assume they do.

Do you still have a duty of confidentiality to your friend? The information is the same, the only thing that has changed is the way in which your friend has told you. A reasonable person is unlikely to consider this a private conversation between the two of you and therefore would not consider this to be a situation obliging you to maintain the confidence of your friend.

There are many ways in which information may be imparted from one person to another, and how the information is imparted is important. In order to tell if the circumstance imparts an obligation of confidentiality on you, ask yourself two questions:

- What does the person imparting the information to you expect you to do with it? Do they expect you to freely share it with others, to share it with a limited number of others, or to keep it confidential?
- Would a reasonable person consider the circumstances in which the information was imparted to you to be one that imposes a duty of confidentiality on you?

If the answer to either or both questions is 'yes' or 'not sure', then an obligation of confidentiality can be implied from the circumstances of the disclosure of information.

Similarly, if a patient tells a healthcare practitioner information in a manner that implies they believe it is in confidence, for example in a private area or as a result of a direct question from a healthcare practitioner, this would suggest an obligation on the part of the healthcare practitioner to treat the information as confidential.

There are times when a patient may ask if they can 'tell you something in confidence'. Because there are times when you have to pass the information on, your response should advise them of that. So, your answer could be, 'yes I will try to keep it confidential, but I may have to pass the information on' (see **Are there occasions when a healthcare practitioner is obliged to disclose confidential patient information? [p. 111]**).

Q What does 'the information must have been divulged to a third person without the permission, and to the detriment, of the person originally communicating it' mean?

A When bringing a case regarding breach of confidentiality, having proved that the information they divulged to a healthcare practitioner had the necessary quality of confidence and was divulged in circumstances that imparted an obligation of confidence on the healthcare practitioner, the third element that a claimant has to prove is that the information was passed to a third party to their detriment.

This requires us to consider who a 'third person' is and what a 'detriment' would be.

DIVULGING INFORMATION TO A THIRD PERSON

If a patient gives some information to a healthcare practitioner, the patient is the first person involved and the healthcare practitioner is the second. A third person would be anyone else who becomes aware of the information. A third person can receive the information either intentionally by being directly told the information or by accident.

Many healthcare practitioners have no intention of deliberately passing on confidential information they have received from a patient and would be horrified to discover that they have accidentally passed this on to a third person. The problem is that accidental disclosure of patient's confidential information is more widespread than we may think or want to believe.

In an observational study in Toronto, Canada in 2002, hospital staff were observed during lift journeys and breaches of patient confidentiality noted when other healthcare practitioners, patients and/or visitors were present. The study identified that patient confidentiality was compromised in over one in ten of the lift journeys (Vigod et al., 2003).

We can make an educated guess that not one of the members of hospital staff intended to breach patient confidentiality. They probably felt safe because they were in their hospital, with colleagues and only sharing information with that colleague. Whatever their intent, patient information was divulged to a third person.

It's not just lift journeys that can lead to an accidental breach of patient confidentiality. Anywhere that a healthcare practitioner feels safe to discuss information with colleagues can pose a potential area for accidental disclosure. This includes hospital canteens and shops; public areas such as hospital entrances and exits where the details of a patient being admitted or discharged may be discussed in the presence of visitors and other patients; and around a nurse's station where patient information is freely discussed whilst other individuals are either passing or waiting to be seen.

Information does not have to be divulged verbally; leaving patient notes in an unattended or insecure publicly accessible place can mean that a non-authorised person will pick up and read those notes. You may not expect someone to pick up a set of patient notes and read them, but they can and do.

Intentional disclosure of patient information includes situations where the healthcare practitioner is attempting to gain some advantage such as selling information on a celebrity patient to a newspaper or magazine. This may occur when the 'celebrity' is still a patient or after they have been discharged, either would be a breach of the duty to the patient.

Many instances of intentional disclosure are not a deliberate breach of confidentiality: the healthcare practitioner intends their action but does not perceive that what they are doing is breaching their patient's confidentiality. We live in an age of the internet and social media. It is so much easier to breach a patient's confidentiality by passing on their information than it used to be.

Consider the group of healthcare practitioners who have a 'selfie' taken because they have just finished a difficult week of work which they publish on one of the photograph hosting sites; the trouble is they don't notice that one member of the group is holding a set of notes where the patient's details are clearly visible. Or the orthopaedic nurse who has a particularly interesting set of x-rays that they want to share for educational purposes on a social media site; only they didn't check whether the patient details were visible before uploading the images. Or the dietician who shares information about a celebrity's strange diet on a social media site and thinks they are fine because they don't mention the celebrity by name; however, they do mention the last project they were involved with and this allows others to identify who the celebrity or person is.

Not one of these healthcare practitioners told a third person information about a patient, yet each will have breached their patient's confidentiality because a third person, in many cases multiple third persons, will have information about their patients.

Unless you are seeking help on a clinical matter, and you must question whether this is the most appropriate method of doing so, posting confidential patient information on a social networking site, or indeed any internet site, even if you believe the information to have been anonymised, is not an acceptable action and should be avoided.

DETRIMENT

A detriment is anything to the disadvantage of the person who provided the information. This could be a financial detriment due to losing their job because of the disclosure of information; the breakup of a relationship due to information that a spouse receives about their partner; loss of opportunity, for example if a celebrity were to stop receiving promotional roles because of information about their past; or reputational loss where a person is perceived differently because information about their sexual history is released to others.

What does 'the information must not be in the public domain already' mean?

Assuming the claimant has proved the first three aspects of their claim, for breach of confidentiality, they then have to prove that the information about them was not already in the public domain.

You may wonder why it is important that the information is not already in the public domain. It is because, if others are already aware of the information, it would be impossible for the claimant to prove that they suffered a detriment because of the healthcare practitioner's breach of confidentiality.

Information is considered to be in the public domain if it is widely known or is freely accessible to others. If information X is known then me telling you X is not a breach of confidentiality.

If the information is not known but is part of a rumour or something that is suspected and the healthcare practitioner confirms that it is true, this can be the necessary action for a breach to be proved as it would not be information in the public domain; it is the confirmation that puts it in the public domain.

Why must it 'be in the public interest to protect the information'?

It is a general legal principle that it must be in the public interest to protect information, otherwise the claimant is unable to claim that the information is confidential and able to form the basis for a claim of breach of confidentiality.

In **Why, as a healthcare practitioner, do I need to know about clinical confidentiality? (p. 97)**, it was noted that clinical confidentiality is necessary in the public interest. This is because clinical confidentiality is needed so that patients will share information freely with their healthcare practitioners.

Does this mean that everything a patient tells a healthcare practitioner is protected in the public interest? No, it doesn't. If every piece of information was protected, this would not be in the public interest as it could mean that other members of society could be placed at risk or harm.

The issue is determining what information is in the public interest to protect and what information does not need to be or should not be protected. The problem is to determine what public interest should have priority when there are competing public interests and when an individual's right to confidentiality trumps public interest and vice versa.

This is something that has been a concern for the Courts, although not always in a healthcare context, it has resulted in some general principles.

CASE NOTE 5.3

D V NATIONAL SOCIETY FOR THE PREVENTION OF CRUELTY TO CHILDREN [1977]

The National Society for the Prevention of Cruelty to Children (NSPCC) received a telephone call from an individual claiming that D's 14-month-old child was being maltreated. An NSPCC inspector immediately visited D's house and found that D's

(Continued)

child had not been maltreated and was in good health. D stated that the visit by the NSPCC inspector had caused her severe clinical depression and wanted to bring a claim against the informant and asked the NSPCC for the name of the informant, but they refused to provide it. Instead D initiated a claim for damages against the NSPCC, alleging that they had been negligent in not checking on the informant before making the inspection visit and as part of that claim asked the court to compel the NSPCC to disclose the identity of the informant so that a claim could be made against them as well.

Although D initially won the right to have the name of the informant released to her, the House of Lords held that to do so would not be in the public interest. This was because, 'the public interest required that those who gave information about child abuse to the society [NSPCC] should be immune from disclosure of their identity in legal proceedings since, otherwise, the society's sources of information would dry up' (D v National Society for the Prevention of Cruelty to Children [1977]: 590).

In 1987 a case was heard that dealt with the issue of publishing information obtained from hospital records in the public interest.

CASE NOTE 5.4

X V Y AND OTHERS [1988]

This case concerned an employee(s) of a health authority who obtained information about two doctors from hospital records and subsequently sold it to a national newspaper. The information was that two practising doctors were being treated for Acquired Immune Deficiency Syndrome (AIDS) at a named hospital. The newspaper had published a general article stating that doctors with AIDS were practising medicine and were intending to publish an article identifying the two doctors on the grounds that it was in the public interest to do so. The health authority was seeking an injunction preventing the newspaper from doing this, also on the grounds of public interest.

The court held that, 'the public interest in preserving the confidentiality of hospital records identified actual or potential AIDS sufferers outweighed the public interest in the freedom of the press to publish such information, because victims of the disease ought not to be deterred by fear of discovery from going to hospital for treatment' (X v Y and others [1988]: 648).

In **What kinds of information might have the 'necessary quality of confidence' or be considered as confidential? (p. 99)**, we examined the Campbell v MGN Limited [2004] case and noted that *The Mirror* newspaper believed that publishing information about Ms Campbell's addiction was in the public interest. The court held that this was not the case.

The point in both of these two cases is that the Courts have identified that there is a difference between what the public may be interested in, which may include celebrity gossip and rumour, and what is in the public interest. The Courts have shown they will uphold the latter but not the former. The main reason for this is that it is not always in the public interest for information from health records to be disclosed as it will restrict individuals from coming forward for treatment.

The following case demonstrates when it is in the public interest to release information obtained from patients.

CASE NOTE 5.5

HUNTER V MANN [1974]

A driver and passengers of a car fled the scene of a road traffic accident. Later that day, a general practitioner (GP) treated a man and, at that man's request, also treated a woman who informed the GP that she had been involved in a motor car accident. The GP advised both of them to contact the police. Some days later, the police asked the GP to provide the names of the man and woman. The GP refused on the grounds that he had obtained the information during a therapeutic relationship and it was therefore confidential. The GP was charged with failing to comply with a requirement under the Road Traffic Act 1972 to provide information which might have led to the identification of the driver who was alleged to be guilty of dangerous driving. The GP was subsequently convicted of this offence and this case was his appeal against that conviction.

It was held that, 'although a doctor was under a duty to his patient not to disclose voluntarily, without the consent of his patient, information which the doctor had gained in his professional capacity' he could be compelled by law to do so (Hunter v Mann [1974]: 414). The public interest in this case to maintain the patient's confidentiality is outweighed by the public interest in identifying individuals involved in road traffic offences.

The public interest in maintaining the confidentiality of information obtained from patients during a therapeutic relationship is a key concept in healthcare law. It is necessary for any patient bringing a claim for breach of confidence to prove that it is in the public interest to maintain confidentiality of that information. However, it is not automatic that protecting a patient's information will always be in the public interest and there is a balancing act to be considered between protecting the rights of the individual and protecting the public interest. As we will see, in the questions that immediately follow, there are times when not only is it permitted (or possible) to share information but times when it must be shared.

How can information be shared without breaching confidentiality?

The obligation upon a healthcare practitioner to maintain the confidentiality of information shared with them by their patients is not absolute. This means that there are circumstances in which it is both lawful and ethical to share the information in the healthcare practitioner's possession.

There are several lawful means of sharing a patient's confidential information with third parties. In this and the five questions that follow, we will explore these means of sharing information. The questions have been written so that the distinction between when a healthcare practitioner *may* share confidential information and when they *should* share that information is made explicit. However, it must be remembered that in practice nothing is straightforward and there may be overlap between the two categories.

As noted in the last few questions, a third party is anyone other than the patient and the healthcare practitioner to whom the patient shared their personal information. When sharing information with a third party, this can be classified into two distinct groups: sharing information with other healthcare practitioners and sharing information with those who are not healthcare practitioners.

Another classification that can be made is when information is shared with the consent of the patient and those occasions when it is shared without the patient's consent.

From what we have discussed so far, it is possible to identify four general situations or circumstances in which a patient's confidential information may be shared with third parties. These are:

- with the patient's consent
- with other healthcare practitioners
- in the best interests of the patient
- in the public interest.

These will be addressed in this question and in the questions that follow.

SHARING INFORMATION WITH THE PATIENT'S CONSENT

The questions on 'Consent' (Chapter 4) clearly show that the patient's valid consent should be obtained before any treatment is provided to them. Consent is one of the fundamental ethical and legal principles in healthcare practice.

If the patient's consent can be obtained for the sharing of their confidential information, this supersedes the healthcare practitioner's duty to maintain confidentiality. It is not possible to breach a duty if you have been absolved from the need to observe the duty. The patient's consent to the sharing of information means that you would not be liable to your employer's disciplinary processes, or a fitness to practise investigation by your regulatory body, and the patient would not be able to sue you for damages relating to the release of information.

It is for this reason that, whenever possible prior to the release of any confidential information, the patient should be asked if they consent to the release of that information. With the valid consent of the patient, information can be released to anyone the patient authorises regardless of whether there is any other legal or ethical justification for doing so.

It is important to remember that, for a healthcare practitioner to be able to rely upon the patient's consent as justification for the release of their confidential information, consent needs to be legally valid. When identifying **What criteria must be fulfilled for consent to be legally valid?** (p. 68), it was noted that there are four legal principles which must be fulfilled for the consent given by the patient to be valid.

If any of these principles are not met, for instance if the healthcare practitioner was pressurising the patient to be able to release their information, the patient's consent to the release of their information would not be legally valid and the healthcare practitioner would not be entitled to rely upon it as justification for the release of the patient's information. However, where the consent is valid, the release of the information can be legally and ethically justified.

SHARING INFORMATION WITH OTHER HEALTHCARE PRACTITIONERS

There is a general expectation that information regarding patients, including confidential information, needs to be and will be shared amongst members of the multidisciplinary healthcare team because of a clinical need; they have to have the information in order to provide care and treatment to the patient. Further to this, it is legally and ethically accepted that patients who consent to healthcare treatment are also giving implied consent for their information, whether confidential or not, to be shared in this way. This is because it is in the patient's best interests that those who are treating them are in possession of relevant clinical information, including any confidential information that is pertinent to the care and treatment the patient requires.

There are limits on sharing information with other healthcare practitioners. These are that:

1. The information should only be shared when there is a genuine clinical need for it to be shared.
2. The information should be limited to those members of the multidisciplinary healthcare team who need it to be able to provide care and treatment to the patient that it concerns.
3. The amount of information that is shared should be limited, so that only that which is strictly necessary to provide care and treatment to the patient is shared.

The principle of implied consent to the sharing of confidential information amongst healthcare practitioners does not extend to those healthcare practitioners who are not members of the patient's multidisciplinary healthcare team. If a healthcare practitioner were to share confidential information about a patient with a fellow healthcare practitioner unconnected with the patient's care and treatment, this would constitute a breach of confidence as it would not constitute a clinical need and therefore is not in the patient's best interests.

SHARING INFORMATION IN THE BEST INTERESTS OF THE PATIENT

There are occasions when, even if they were asked, patients would not be able to provide consent for the sharing of the information; as they are not considered competent. In these circumstances, the legal principles that govern the treatment are based on acting in the patient's best interests. Sharing information, even confidential information, that is clinically relevant with other members of the patient's multidisciplinary healthcare team would be in their best interests.

Thus, confidential information of adult patients who are incompetent can be shared with other healthcare practitioners. This is provided that the information being shared is relevant to the patient's care and treatment, and the information that is shared is limited to that which is needed for the members of the multidisciplinary healthcare team to undertake their individual roles in caring and treating the patient.

Acting in the patient's best interests by sharing confidential information is something that will be revisited in the questions below while considering when information should be divulged in the patient's best interests.

See further discussion on sharing information in the best interests of the patient in **Are there occasions when a healthcare practitioner is obliged to disclose confidential patient information? (p. 111).**

Q Is it OK to share information that has been anonymised?

A This is a question that has been considered in the Court of Appeal in recent years.

CASE NOTE 5.6

R V DEPARTMENT OF HEALTH, EX PARTE SOURCE INFORMATICS LTD [2000]

Source Informatics Ltd was a database company that wanted to obtain data from pharmacists regarding general practitioner (GP) prescriptions for which the pharmacists were going to be paid. This data was to consist of the name of the GP and the name and quantity of the drug prescribed. The data was not to include patient names. On learning of this, The Department of Health issued guidance which stated that a duty of confidence would still be owed to patients even if data were anonymised. Source Informatics Ltd asked for the Department of Health guidance to be reviewed by the court as they believed that the sharing of anonymised information would not breach the confidentiality of patients.

Based on the judgment in the Court of Appeal case, if data concerning a patient is suitably anonymised, so that the patient cannot be identified, it would not be unlawful for that data to be shared.

The challenge in anonymising data is in having the data truly anonymised so that no features remain which could identify a specific individual.

Are there occasions when a healthcare practitioner is obliged to disclose confidential patient information?

As noted when considering **How can information be shared without breaching confidentiality? (p. 108)**, the healthcare practitioner's duty of confidentiality is not absolute. Indeed, as well as circumstances in which the healthcare practitioner may share information, there are circumstances in which the healthcare practitioner is obliged to do so, and it is those we will consider here.

SHARING INFORMATION IN THE BEST INTERESTS OF THE PATIENT

Although this point was discussed in **How can information be shared without breaching confidentiality? (p. 108)**, it is necessary to consider the best interests of the patient here from another perspective.

We have already seen that confidential information can be disclosed to a third party without the patient's consent when it is in the patient's best interests to do so, for instance if the patient is incompetent and so unable to provide consent.

Another way in which the best interests of the patient can be used to justify disclosure of confidential information is when the healthcare practitioner suspects the patient may have been or may be subject to abuse or neglect.

In situations such as these, whether the patient is an adult or child, the healthcare practitioner has a duty to the patient to protect them from further mistreatment. In the case of a competent adult, this may be limited to advising and supporting the patient; without their consent, no other action can be taken.

For incompetent adults and children, the healthcare practitioner may need to inform a third party of their suspicions. Whenever possible the healthcare practitioner should obtain the patient's consent to disclose information regarding the suspected mistreatment. Where this is not possible, either because the patient will not consent or to seek the patient's consent may put them at risk of harm or mean that they leave the healthcare practitioner's care, the healthcare practitioner's duty to protect their patient will supersede their duty of confidentiality to the patient. Informing a third party may also be appropriate where a competent adult consents.

Where a healthcare practitioner needs to act in the best interests of the patient to protect them by disclosing confidential information to a third party, they should disclose the minimum information that is necessary for the third party to take appropriate action and inform the third party whether the patient has consented to the disclosure or, if not, whether the patient is aware of the disclosure. Disclosure to a third party has to be to a relevant authority that will be able to act on the patient's behalf in relation to the suspected mistreatment, such as social services or the police.

SHARING INFORMATION IN THE PUBLIC INTEREST

As well as disclosing information in the best interests of the patient, disclosure of confidential information may also be required in the public interest.

There is not a single entity that is the 'public interest'. Rather, there is a set of circumstances and principles, which place an obligation upon the healthcare practitioner to disclose confidential patient information, that are said to have a benefit not for the patient but for a third party or parties, the elusive public interest.

Disclosure of confidential patient information in the public interest is not something that should be undertaken lightly and any healthcare practitioner considering doing so needs to consider the full circumstances relevant to their particular context.

In the case of Attorney-General v Guardian Newspapers (No 2) [1990] (see **What are the principles of clinical confidentiality? [p. 99]**), it was found that there is a balancing act between the public interest in maintaining and protecting patient confidentiality and the public interest in disclosure. It was noted that the starting point for considering the public interest was in maintaining confidentiality and only when there is a compelling need for disclosure that overrides this should disclosure be made.

Some of the strong and compelling reasons that may be said to require disclosure in the public interest include:

- child or vulnerable person protection
- to protect third parties
- statutory requirements
- public health requirements
- police investigations
- prevention of crime.

The protection of children and vulnerable persons has been discussed above when considering the best interests of the patient and so won't be explored any further, except to say that where a healthcare practitioner believes there is a possibility that a child or a vulnerable person is being abused by their patient, they must disclose this information in order to protect the child or vulnerable person.

A healthcare practitioner may be required to disclose a patient's confidential information in the public interest to protect a third party. This is known as a 'duty to warn'. Because there are particular conditions when disclosure may be made as a duty to warn, this will be considered more fully in the question on duty to warn that follows.

Several Acts of Parliament place a statutory obligation upon a healthcare practitioner that either permits or obligates them to disclose confidential information. Examples of these statutory obligations include:

- Abortion Act 1967 – which requires details regarding the termination of pregnancies to be reported to the relevant authority.
- Misuse of Drugs Act 1971 – which requires doctors to supply certain information relating to the treatment of patients addicted to controlled drugs.
- Public Health (Control of Disease) Act 1984 – which requires that, if a healthcare practitioner is aware of the patient with certain notifiable diseases, they are required to inform the relevant authority.
- Road Traffic Act 1988 – requires that information that identifies a driver of a vehicle who has committed certain offences under the Act is provided when requested.

An example of a disclosure of confidential information made as a public health requirement in the public interest would be where a healthcare practitioner was aware of a patient with a highly transmissible infectious disease who will not accept treatment or attend hospital. The healthcare practitioner would be justified in informing the relevant authorities of the patient's details in order that the patient could be conveyed to hospital and/or receive treatment to prevent the patient from posing further risk to the public.

Healthcare practitioners have no general obligation to assist the police with their enquiries. This means that there is no need to automatically disclose confidential information that would be useful to the police. However, there are certain circumstances under which healthcare practitioners are required to assist the police such as the Road Traffic Act 1988.

The Road Traffic Act 1988 supersedes the Road Traffic Act 1972 and it was this Act which was used to convict the doctor in the Hunter v Mann [1974] case, which we discussed when we considered **Why must it 'be in the public interest to protect the information'?** (p. 105).

Another occasion when the healthcare practitioner has an obligation to provide information to the police would be under the Terrorism Act 2000, in relation to a patient involved or suspected of being involved in terrorist activities.

It is not the role of the healthcare practitioner to investigate crime, but they should not obstruct the police and their investigations. It would not constitute obstruction to fail to answer the police if the police questions were in relation to confidential information and there is no lawful justification for the healthcare practitioner to disclose this.

The situation can be said to change if the healthcare practitioner is aware that their patient may be involved in criminal activity, the crime is one of a grave nature and, without the healthcare practitioner's information, the prevention or detection of the crime may be hindered. In this situation, the healthcare practitioner may disclose the information they possess to the relevant authority, which may be the police, in the public interest. This aspect of disclosing information in the public interest is discussed in **What is a duty to warn? (p. 114).**

Even where no other public interest justification exists for the disclosure of confidential information, a healthcare practitioner may find themselves compelled to disclose their information. This would occur where a court of law requires them to do so, including as a witness before the court. The therapeutic relationship is no protection against disclosing information when requested to do so by a court. If requested by a court to provide confidential patient information, you should do so. In fact, failure to disclose information to the court, when requested to do so, could lead you to being found in contempt of court and subject to the court's punishment.

Other examples of disclosing confidential information in the public interest would include informing the Driver and Vehicle Licensing Agency (DVLA) that a patient was unfit to drive where they cannot be persuaded to stop driving, or to contact the DVLA themselves.

It is important to note that, when disclosure of confidential patient information is made in the public interest, it has to be made to the relevant authority. Otherwise, there is still the potential for a breach of confidence to exist. For instance, in relation to a patient who is unfit to drive, the disclosure would be to the DVLA and not the patient's relatives or their insurer. It is the DVLA who is responsible for deciding who is fit to drive and has the power to suspend a driving licence or take appropriate steps with regard to the patient's driving.

In summary, where there is a legal or ethical justification for the disclosure of confidential patient information, in the public interest or the best interests of the patient, you may disclose necessary information to the appropriate authority. Where the legal or ethical justification does not exist, you shouldn't disclose the information.

When confidential information about a patient is disclosed without the patient's consent, whenever possible the patient should be informed of the disclosure and the reason for it.

Q **What is a duty to warn?**

A When considering the occasions when a healthcare practitioner can be obliged to divulge confidential information they have received from a patient to a third person, one of the reasons put forward was when a duty to warn exists.

A duty to warn exists when the healthcare practitioner has received information which indicates that there is a risk of serious harm to others. The duty is to warn the third person of the risk to them or to ensure that an appropriate individual is warned of the risk so that they can take the relevant action. Two cases illustrate how the duty to warn operates in practice, so that third parties may be protected by the disclosure of confidential information.

CASE NOTE 5.7

TARASOFF V REGENTS OF THE UNIVERSITY OF CALIFORNIA [1976]

This is an American case where a male patient, Prosenjit Poddar, informed his psychologist, Dr Moore, that he intended to kill Tatiana Tarasoff, with whom he was infatuated and who had spurned his advances. Dr Moore had had several sessions with Mr Poddar and it was during the seventh that the intention to harm Miss Tarasoff was disclosed. Dr Moore duly contacted the police and alerted them to what Mr Poddar had disclosed to him. The police briefly detained Mr Poddar but released him when he promised to stay away from Ms Tarasoff.

At no time was a warning given to Miss Tarasoff informing her of the risk from Mr Poddar, which would have allowed her to take action to protect herself from the possibility of attack. Mr Poddar subsequently attacked and killed Ms Tarasoff.

The case was brought by Miss Tarasoff's parents who were suing Dr Moore and the police for the failure to warn Ms Tarasoff of the danger that Mr Poddar posed to her. Miss Tarasoff's parents won the case as the California Supreme Court held that Dr Moore owed a duty of care to Miss Tarasoff and had breached this duty by failing to warn her of the danger she was facing.

The judgment in the Tarasoff case means that the normal therapeutic privilege between a patient and their healthcare practitioner which encompasses the duty of confidentiality ends when the healthcare practitioner is aware of a specific risk of serious harm to an identifiable person from their patient. In these circumstances, the healthcare practitioner has a duty to warn the identified individual even if this involves breaching their patient's confidentiality.

The Tarasoff case is an American case and as such does not directly contribute to the law in the United Kingdom. However, an English case has considered the duty to warn, including the Tarasoff judgment, and reached a similar judgment.

CASE NOTE 5.8

W V EGDELL AND OTHERS [1990]

W had shot seven people, killing five and wounding two, and was detained in a secure hospital. It was known that W had an interest in firearms and explosives. W applied to be discharged or transferred to a regional secure unit; this could be a step towards eventual discharge. W's application was opposed by the Secretary of State.

(Continued)

In order to support his application, W's solicitors appointed an independent consultant psychiatrist, Dr Egdell, to provide a report on his mental state. This was completed and sent to W's solicitors. However, Dr Egdell's report strongly opposed any transfer, noting W's long-standing interest in firearms and explosives, and recommended further tests and treatment, including that W remained a danger to the public. In view of Dr Egdell's report, W withdrew his application.

Because W withdrew his application, Dr Egdell's report would not be seen by those overseeing W's clinical management. When Dr Egdell learned that his report would not be seen by the tribunal or those overseeing W, concerned that they would not have a full picture of the risk that W posed, he arranged for the medical director of the secure hospital and the Secretary of State to receive copies.

Later W was due to have his case reconsidered as part of the automatic review process carried out under the Mental Health Act 1983. The Secretary of State sent a copy of Dr Egdell's report to the tribunal when referring W's case to them.

When W learnt that the report had been disclosed, he applied to the court for an injunction to prevent anyone using or disclosing the report, for all copies of the report to be sent to him and for damages relating to breach of confidence.

The court dismissed W's claim on the basis that, although Dr Egdell owed a duty of confidence to W, that confidence was subordinate to the duty that Dr Egdell had to the public to ensure that the relevant authorities were fully informed about W's mental condition when making any decisions about W's treatment and his future so that they could make an informed judgement.

What these cases show is that there can be competing interests on the healthcare practitioner's duty: between the duty to the patient and the duty to the public. In normal circumstances, the duty of confidence to the patient will outweigh that to the public. However, where a clear risk of serious harm exists to an identifiable individual or the public at large, that is a continuing risk and not one that has passed, the duty to warn supersedes the duty of confidence owed to the patient. It is also worth noting that the judgments in these cases indicate that the duty to warn exists when others are at risk of harm, not when it is the patient themselves who is at risk.

It is worth contrasting the Egdell case with that of Campbell v MGN Limited [2004] (see **What kinds of information might have the 'necessary quality of confidence' or be considered as confidential? [p. 99]**) to see what the Courts consider to be in the public interest.

In the Egdell case, based upon Dr Egdell's report, there was a clear risk of serious harm to the public by W and it was therefore in the public interest for them to be made aware of this risk so that measures could be taken to protect them. Whereas in the Campbell case, there was no risk to the public and no need to protect them from Ms Campbell's actions. Rather, the information about Ms Campbell's drug use is something that the public can be said to be interested in rather than something that is in the public interest.

Q Where there is a duty to warn, who should be told?

A There is a conflict between the competing duties of the healthcare practitioner to their patients and to the public in general. In managing these duties, a healthcare practitioner needs to ensure that any disclosures they make are lawful and are made to the appropriate person or agency.

In the W v Egdell and others [1990] case (see **What is a duty to warn? [p. 114]**), the disclosure of the report was made to the medical director of the secure hospital and the Secretary of State who subsequently disclosed it to the tribunal. Both individuals were in a position to influence the decisions being made about W in the public interest.

The duty to warn does not mean that the healthcare practitioner has a right to disclose their patient's confidential information to anyone because this fulfils the duty. The disclosure needs to be to the minimum number of appropriate people or agencies in order that the public interest can be protected.

It would seem obvious that, if identified individuals are at risk, they can be informed of the risk even if that means disclosing confidential information. Likewise, if necessary for public protection, the police or similar agencies can be informed. The aim of the disclosure is the public interest by which is meant public protection. Therefore, if Dr Egdell had chosen to contact a newspaper and provide them with confidential information regarding W instead of those he did provide the report to, it is most likely that he would have been found in breach of confidentiality as this would not have been an appropriate way for him to protect the public.

Essentially, this can be summed up as only disclosing to those who have a legitimate need to know.

Q What can be disclosed when fulfilling a duty to warn?

A The minimum amount of confidential information that is needed to protect the public. This means only that which it is absolutely necessary to disclose in the public interest. Anything that can be safely withheld should be.

We can consider the case of a patient (A) who has made a specific threat towards an identifiable individual (B) during outpatient psychiatric treatment to a healthcare practitioner (C).

Assuming that A poses a serious risk of harm to B that is real and immediate, C could legitimately warn B of the risk and the type of risk and also that the risk is from A. There would most likely be no benefit in C informing B of A's past medical history or their current diagnosis. Similarly, it would be unlikely that C could inform B of the current medication that A is taking. This is because these additional pieces of information would be unlikely to help B in reducing their personal risk.

If C chose to inform the police of the risk A posed to B then some of this additional information, for instance A's diagnosis, may be relevant in enabling the police to assist B.

In either case, disclosing information to B or to the police, the disclosure is to someone who is able to address the risk and the information disclosed is necessary to assist them in doing this.

 If a patient is concerned about their confidentiality being breached, what remedies are available to them?

A If the patient is concerned that their confidential information may be breached because of the way that their health records are being stored or the lack of storage, or because of the way that patient information is discussed in public areas; the patient would have the right to bring this to the attention of someone in a senior position and ask them to address the issue.

There are two possible legal remedies that the patient has available to them: which one is used is dependent upon whether the patient's confidential information has been publicly disclosed or if it is about to be disclosed.

Where the information has yet to be publicly disclosed, the remedy available to the patient is an injunction. An injunction is an order of a court which orders someone, or an organisation, to refrain from a particular act. With regards to confidentiality, the injunction would order someone not to publish the information relating to the patient. If the person continues to do the act prohibited by the injunction, for instance by publishing the information about the patient, they would be in contempt of court and subject to a penalty from that court. The penalty could be an unlimited fine or a jail sentence of up to two years.

As well as preventing the release of information, an injunction can also be used to prevent further publication. For instance, if the patient's information has been published on a particular website but a newspaper was intending to publish it, an injunction could be issued to the website to remove it and also a separate injunction to the newspaper to prevent it from being published again.

The problem that a patient concerned about their confidentiality would have is in knowing that someone intended to breach their confidentiality by publishing their personal information. If the patient was not aware of the intention to publish their personal information, they would be unable to apply for an injunction to prevent this.

Breaches of confidentiality are final in that it is not possible to undo the breach; once the information is publicly known, it cannot be unknown. Therefore, where the patient's confidential information has been published, the remedy available to them is to seek damages from those who published the confidential information. The patient, in seeking damages, would have to prove that they have suffered some form of loss. It is unlikely that the loss would be monetary and is more likely to be a form of embarrassment or loss of status and injury to feelings. This becomes difficult to quantify and for adequate damages to be awarded. In the Campbell v MGN Limited [2004] (see **What kinds of information might have the 'necessary quality of confidence' or be considered** as confidential? [p. 99]), it is notable that the damages awarded to Ms Campbell were only £3,500 in total.

The damages awarded are payable by those who are deemed to have breached the patient's confidentiality. In a case where a healthcare practitioner provides information to a newspaper for money, damages would be payable by both the healthcare practitioner and the newspaper, in proportion to their culpability determined by the court.

The patient would also be able to raise a complaint with the relevant hospital or clinic where the healthcare practitioner worked, and to bring to the attention of the relevant healthcare regulatory body as a fitness to practise issue due to the healthcare practitioner's breach of their code of conduct.

Q
A

What are Caldicott Guardians and how do they relate to confidentiality?

'Caldicott Guardian' is a common term seen in many forms of literature that deal with patient information and confidentiality, and in National Health Service (NHS) and Department of Health documents. The term is so ubiquitous that it is seldom defined.

In 1997 a report was published by the Department of Health, which was based upon a review that had been commissioned by the Chief Medical Officer due to concerns about the way in which patient information was being used within the NHS. Its full title is *Report on the Review of Patient-Identifiable Information* (Department of Health, 1997), but it is generally referred to as the 'Caldicott Report' after the name of the person chairing the committee, Dame Fiona Caldicott. As the Report notes, 'such concern was largely due to development of information technology in the service, and its capacity to disseminate information about patients rapidly and extensively' (Department of Health, 1997: i).

The Caldicott Committee made 16 recommendations in the Report concerning how patient information should be managed. Recommendation number 3 was that, 'a senior person, preferably a health professional, should be nominated in each health organisation to act as a guardian, responsible for safeguarding the confidentiality of patient information' (Department of Health, 1997: iv). When this recommendation was subsequently implemented, these individuals became known as 'Caldicott Guardians'.

Caldicott Guardians are a mandatory requirement for all NHS organisations and local authorities providing social services. There is a national body of Caldicott Guardians in the United Kingdom, known as the UK Caldicott Guardian Council (its website is available at: www.ukcgc.uk/).

An organisation's Caldicott Guardian is responsible for overseeing how confidential information is managed and protected within the organisation. The UK Caldicott Guardian Council states in its manual that the responsibilities of a Caldicott Guardian are fourfold, as follows:

Strategy & governance: the Caldicott Guardian should champion confidentiality issues at Board/senior management team level, should sit on an organisation's Information Governance Board/Group and act as both the 'conscience' of the organisation and as an enabler for appropriate information sharing.

Confidentiality & data protection expertise: the Caldicott Guardian should develop a strong knowledge of confidentiality and data protection matters, drawing upon support staff working within an organisation's Caldicott and information governance functions, but also on external sources of advice and guidance where available.

Internal information processing: the Caldicott Guardian should ensure that confidentiality issues are appropriately reflected in organisational strategies, policies and working procedures for staff. The key areas of work that need to be addressed by the organisation's Caldicott function are detailed in the Information Governance Toolkit.

Information sharing: the Caldicott Guardian should oversee all arrangements, protocols and procedures where confidential personal information may be shared with external bodies and others with responsibilities for social care and safeguarding. This includes flows of information to and from partner agencies, sharing through IT systems, disclosure for research, and disclosure to the police. (The UK Caldicott Guardian Council, 2020).

The UK Caldicott Guardian Council also notes that staff working within organisations should be encouraged to seek assistance from their Caldicott Guardian if they have concerns or need advice regarding confidentiality or issues relating to patients' personal information.

As a healthcare practitioner, do I need to know about the Data Protection Act 2018?

The Data Protection Act 2018 came into force on 25th May 2018 and repealed the Data Protection Act 1998. It was the legislation which implemented the General Data Protection Regulation 2016/679/EU (known as GDPR) into UK law.

The Act applies to personal information and this includes health records, whether in paper or electronic form. The Act is very long with over 200 sections and 20 schedules and does not make for light reading; the main point to note is that there are six data protection principles contained within the Act. These principles are:

- processing of personal data must be lawful, fair and transparent
- personal data must be processed for specified legitimate purposes
- personal data must not be excessive in relation to the purpose for which it is held
- personal data must be accurate and up to date

- personal data must be kept no longer than is necessary
- personal data must be processed in such a way that it is secure.

The Act contains penalties for those who breach its provisions.

Whilst you need to be aware of the general principles of the Data Protection Act 2018, if you abide by the ethical, legal and regulatory guidance regarding confidentiality you should not fall foul of it.

Q

Do any of the principles of confidentiality change if my patient is under 18?

A

When discussing **Are children able to consent to their own treatment? (p. 82)**, it was noted that someone under the age of 18 is legally considered a child but that someone aged 16–18 is considered competent to be able to consent on their own behalf, whilst those under the age of 16 have to prove they are competent to consent.

It is easy to imagine situations where the treatment of a person under the age of 18 will involve a particular issue relating to confidentiality. Indeed, the case that established the right of a child under the age of 16 to consent on their own behalf in certain circumstances, Gillick v West Norfolk and Wisbech Area Health Authority and another [1985] (see **Are children able to consent to their own treatment? [p. 82]**), concerned whether a child was able to receive contraceptive advice and treatment without the knowledge of their parents.

When considering confidentiality issues in patients under the age of 18, the starting point is to consider whether the child who is your patient has the capacity and competence to make their own treatment decisions.

As said above, where the child is between the ages of 16 and 18, they have the legal right afforded to them, under the Family Law Reform Act 1969, Section 8, to consent on their own behalf. If they are legally entitled to provide their own consent, it follows they are legally entitled to make their own decisions regarding confidentiality and should be treated as an adult in these matters.

The right of a child under the age of 16 to confidentiality was considered in the Axon case.

CASE NOTE 5.9

R (ON THE APPLICATION OF AXON) V SECRETARY OF STATE FOR HEALTH AND ANOTHER [2006]

Sue Axon applied to the court for a declaration that a doctor was not obliged to keep confidential contraceptive, sexually transmitted disease or abortion advice and treatment

(Continued)

that they proposed to provide to a child. Further, that they must not provide that advice and treatment without the knowledge of the parents. The court rejected Mrs Axon's application, holding that there is no obligation on a medical practitioner to inform a young person's parents or to ensure that they were informed about proposed advice or treatment in relation to contraception, sexually transmitted disease or abortion. It was noted that in making this judgment the court was upholding the principle established in the Gillick v West Norfolk and Wisbech Area Health Authority and another [1985] case.

For those patients under the age of 16, competence is based on the healthcare practitioner's assessment of whether the child has the intellectual and emotional maturity to make a decision regarding their own condition and treatment. As noted above, this is based upon the judgment in the Gillick case. Where a child is judged to be able to make decisions and provide consent regarding their own condition and treatment, they are referred to as 'Gillick competent'. A 'Gillick competent' child has the same rights as anyone else who is competent to make their own decisions and provide their own consent. Therefore, they can expect the same duty of confidentiality to be available to them as to any other competent patient.

It is naturally possible for a patient under the age of 16 to be considered to be 'Gillick competent' for some procedures but not for others; this being dependent upon the child's understanding and maturity regarding the treatment being proposed.

Discussions regarding disclosure of a child's confidential information should not be based upon the child's age but upon whether the information needs to be disclosed in the public interest or whether there is some other lawful reason for the disclosure of the confidential information, or it is in the child's best interests for the information to be disclosed such as where abuse is suspected.

Any confidential information that is released, either in the child's best interests or in the public interest, must only be disclosed to individuals on a need to know basis to the minimum number of people, and limited to only the information that it is absolutely necessary to release to achieve the purpose of the child's or public interest.

Do any of the principles of confidentiality change after the death of the patient?

The healthcare practitioner's duty to maintain their patient's confidentiality does not end with the death of the patient.

Actions for breach of confidentiality pass to the estate of the individual upon their death. This means that the healthcare practitioner is not able to sell a story to the media about a celebrity patient of theirs once that celebrity has died. This is because, as well as the possibility of disciplinary action by their employer and a fitness to practise investigation by the relevant healthcare regulatory body, there would still be the possibility of facing a claim for damages for breach of confidence;

although the estate of the individual would have to prove that it has suffered some loss caused by the breach of confidentiality.

On a patient's death, their confidential information does not pass to the estate of the deceased but rather remains confidential.

It is possible that, after a patient's death, a spouse or other relative of the deceased may contact a healthcare practitioner and ask for specific information that ordinarily would be confidential. This can put the healthcare practitioner in a dilemma. If the patient were alive, they could be asked if they consent to the release of information; as they are dead, this is not possible. Instead, the healthcare practitioner needs to consider what the patient would want them to do, that is what is in the deceased patient's best interests.

If the patient had made a specific request or statement prior to their death that, under no circumstances whatsoever would they want anyone to know a particular piece of information, it is difficult to see how disclosing that information could be in their best interests. However, most individuals do not make such statements or requests before their death and this calls for a judgement to be made by the healthcare practitioner.

It is possible to take a pragmatic view based on whether the information requested would assist the individual in any way or if knowing that information could affect how they remember the deceased relative. From a legal perspective, one can ask if the information were disclosed, who would complain or bring a legal case for breach of confidentiality; however, this still leaves the ethical dilemma of whether to release information or not. A healthcare practitioner placed in this situation needs to proceed on the basis of what they consider would be in the patient's best interests based on their knowledge of the patient.

Sharing patient information after their death is discussed further in **What happens to health records after a patient's death? (p. 152).**

Does research in the healthcare setting raise any special issues in relation to confidentiality?

Some healthcare practitioners will be more involved with research than others; whilst some healthcare practitioners may make primary research the focus of their careers. However, if we consider research in its widest sense to include teaching, internal and external audit, primary and secondary research, then all healthcare practitioners will at some point during their training and practice be involved in research activity.

The first point that needs to be made is that the general principles of confidentiality discussed in response to the questions above still need to be considered when undertaking research in the healthcare setting. This means that information obtained from patients should be treated as confidential and only be used for the purpose for which it was given.

In the research context, information from patients as research participants can be provided consensually or non-consensually. Obtaining information consensually is always the preferred option when it is possible to do so. This means obtaining valid consent from the patient as a research participant to use their personal information in research. It doesn't matter if the information being obtained from the patient for the purposes of the research is directly healthcare related or not.

Sometimes it is not possible to obtain consent from the patient to use their information in a research study. Such circumstances may include research that involves historical data and research where the subject group may be incompetent to consent, for example research involving sedated patients in intensive care units. As patient information being collected as data is not going to be used for the individual's care, it is not possible to use the best interests principle instead of consent.

In these circumstances, wherever possible, the patient information should be anonymised so that individual patients cannot be identified either from the data itself or from the report that is written based upon that data.

Whenever research is being undertaken with human subjects, ethical approval needs to be sought from a research ethics committee, or similar. Research ethics committees can be located within NHS Trusts, universities and at regional and national level. The NHS has an executive non-departmental public body known as the NHS Health Research Authority, established under the provisions of the Care Act 2014, which oversees research ethics committees reviewing health and social care research in England.

Seeking approval for a research project can sometimes seem to involve cumbersome processes before approval can be obtained; though it must be remembered that the role of the research ethics committee is protection of the subjects, this includes their rights, dignity, safety and wellbeing as well as promoting and facilitating research that is of benefit to society. This is why they require the researcher to provide detailed information about what information will be collected, how it will be used and what information will be provided to the research participant.

Research ethics committees expect the researcher to abide by ethical codes for research. Where consent cannot be obtained from research subjects, the reason for this will need to be justified along with how the information collected will be stored safely as well as how the identity of the individuals concerned will be protected.

In situations where consent cannot be obtained and anonymisation of the data is not achievable, it is still possible to receive ethical approval for the research undertaken but additional safeguards may be expected or required.

There is a possibility that retrospective consent may be allowed when information needs to be obtained when the patient is unable to consent; this is then stored until permission to use the data can be obtained from the patient. Details regarding storage and protection of the data whilst being stored will need to be provided to the research ethics committee.

Some research projects may have a legitimate reason to identify certain locations where identifying these areas, such as the use of postcodes, could lead to identification of individuals. Unless consent can be obtained from the individuals for their postcodes to be used, this should only be undertaken once ethical approval has been sought and granted.

As well as providing review and approval of potential research projects, research ethics committees can also provide advice and guidance regarding suitable methods for the collection of personal information to be used as data on specific projects.

Approval for research projects needs to be obtained before the research project commences. As well as approval from a research ethics committee, the permission of an employer will be needed before patients can be approached regarding the obtaining and use of their information for research projects.

If you are in any doubt whatsoever as to whether you can use a patient's information in a research context, do not use the information before you have obtained approval to do so.

  Does my duty of confidentiality to my patients end when I move employers or when I cease being a healthcare practitioner?

The healthcare practitioner's duty to maintain their patient's confidentiality is not related solely to their employment by a specific employer. Although the employer will have an expectation that the healthcare practitioner will uphold their duty of confidentiality to the patients in their care, and this is likely to feature in a contract of employment, this is not the only influence on the healthcare practitioner regarding confidentiality. As noted in the questions above, the duty of confidentiality arises from the common law and statutory law, as well as from obligations based on registration with one of the healthcare regulatory bodies. As such, the duty of confidentiality owed by the healthcare practitioner to the patient does not end if the healthcare practitioner changes employer.

Similarly, if the healthcare practitioner retires or changes their occupation to a non-healthcare related field, the duty of confidentiality to their former patients does not end. Although they would cease registration with their healthcare regulatory body and this would mean that the regulatory body would be unable to hold a fitness to practise investigation, all the other legal remedies available to someone whose confidence has been breached would still be available to any past patient of the former healthcare practitioner.

In short, a change of employer or career, or retirement, does not end the duty of confidentiality that a healthcare practitioner or former healthcare practitioner owes to their past patients.

  As a brief review, what are the reasons or ways in which confidential information may be shared with third parties?

The duty to maintain confidentiality is not absolute. There are five main ways in which confidential patient information may be disclosed. These are:

- when the patient consents to their information being shared; this consent can be express or implied
- when the information is shared with other healthcare practitioners who are involved in the care or treatment of the patient and need that information to be able to provide that care or treatment
- in the best interests of the patient – either when the patient is incompetent and unable to provide consent, or when obtaining consent is not possible because of the need to protect the patient
- in the public interest, this includes statutory requirements to disclose information, when ordered to do so by a court, and when there is a duty to warn others. If the confidential information needs to be shared due to a legal requirement to do so, either statutory or common law, then no breach of confidentiality will occur on disclosure to the appropriate authority
- when the information has been suitably anonymised so that the patient is not identifiable from that information. Although it could be argued that, strictly speaking, this is not confidential information as it cannot be traced back to an identifiable person.

SUMMARY

- Any patient information that you come across in the course of your duties as a healthcare practitioner is confidential information. As such, it should not be repeated to a third person without the consent of the person who supplied the information to you, except in very limited and specific circumstances.
- Confidentiality is a deeply held principle of healthcare practice.
- Confidentiality exists both for the protection of patients and the public, and is essential in ensuring that patient information can be shared in ways that are both timely and lawful.
- Patients provide information in the knowledge and expectation that it will only be used for their benefit and will not be shared unnecessarily or with just anyone.
- The legal and ethical principles of confidentiality are relatively simple; it is their application in practice that can cause uncertainty and confusion.
- All healthcare practitioners have a duty of confidentiality to their patients.
- To be capable of being confidential, the information must:
  - have a quality of confidence
  - not already be in the public domain
  - have been imparted to a healthcare practitioner in circumstances which suggest an obligation on the healthcare practitioner
  - it must be in the public interest to protect it.
- The duty to maintain confidentiality is not absolute.
- Information can be shared without breaching confidentiality with the patient's consent, with other healthcare practitioners using the patient's implied consent, or in the best interests of the patient.

- Personal information that is truly anonymised so that no features remain which could identify a specific individual can be shared without being a breach of the duty of confidentiality.
- There are certain circumstances in which it is necessary to share confidential information even if the patient will not consent to its sharing. These include:
  o protection of children or vulnerable persons
  o to protect third parties
  o statutory requirements
  o public health requirements
  o police investigations
  o prevention of crime.
- A duty to warn individuals of a specific risk of harm to them exists as part of the public interest.
- The duty to warn must be made to appropriate individuals or agencies and should be the minimum amount of information that will fulfil the duty.
- There are several remedies available to someone who is concerned that their personal information is being shared.
- Caldicott Guardians exist in NHS organisations and local authorities to oversee the management of confidential information in those organisations.
- The provisions within the Data Protection Act 2018 extend to health records.
- The duty of confidentiality extends to those under the age of 18.
- The duty of confidentiality does not end on the death of the patient.
- Research with patients raises special issues in relation to confidentiality such as the need to obtain ethical approval and consent from patients.
- A change of employer or career, or retirement, does not end the duty of confidentiality that a healthcare practitioner or former healthcare practitioner owes to their past patients.

REFERENCES

Abortion Act 1967.
Attorney-General v Guardian Newspapers (No 2) [1990] 1 AC 109.
Campbell v MGN Limited [2004] UKHL 22.
Care Act 2014.
Coco v Clark [1968] FSR 415.
Cornock, M. and Nichols, A. (2008) 'Caught on camera', *Nursing Standard, 23*(5): 64.
D v National Society for the Prevention of Cruelty to Children [1977] 1 All ER 589.
Data Protection Act 2018.
Department of Health (1997) *Report on the Review of Patient-Identifiable Information.* Department of Health: London.
Department of Health (2003) *Confidentiality: NHS Code of Practice.* Department of Health: London.
Family Law Reform Act 1969.
General Data Protection Regulation 2016/679/EU.
Gillick v West Norfolk and Wisbech Area Health Authority and another [1985] 3 ALL ER 402.

Health and Social Care Act 2012.

Human Rights Act 1998.

Hunter v Mann [1974] 2 All ER 414.

Kennedy, I. and Grubb, A. (eds) (1998) *Principles of Medical Law*. Oxford University Press: Oxford.

Mental Health Act 1983.

Misuse of Drugs Act 1971

National Health Service Act 2006.

Public Health (Control of Disease) Act 1984.

R v Department of Health, ex parte Source Informatics Ltd [2000] 1 All ER 786.

R (on the application of Axon) v Secretary of State for Health and another [2006] EWHC 37 (Admin).

Road Traffic Act 1972.

Road Traffic Act 1988.

Stephens v Avery [1998] 2 All ER 477.

Tarasoff v Regents of the University of California (1976) 131 Cal Rptr 14.

Terrorism Act 2000.

The UK Caldicott Guardian Council (2020) *A Manual for Caldicott Guardians*. Available at: www.ukcgc.uk/manual/contents.

Vigod, S., Bell, C. and Bohnen, J. (2003) 'Privacy of patients' information in hospital lifts: observational study', *British Medical Journal*, vol. 327: 1024–5.

W v Egdell and others [1990] 1 All ER 835.

X v Y and others [1988] 2 All ER 648.

HEALTH RECORDS

This chapter explores what a health record is and the purpose for which it is made. It also considers practical issues such as how an entry is made in a health record, the standard required for making an entry, and the use of jargon and abbreviations. It reflects upon how a health record may be used and accessed, by the patient and by others.

In this chapter, 'health record' will be used as shorthand for any documentation that a healthcare practitioner needs to complete and maintain.

QUESTIONS COVERED IN CHAPTER 6

- What is a health record?
- What is the purpose of a health record?
- Who owns and controls a health record?
- What problems can arise with a health record?
- Is there a standard, either legal or regulatory, I have to reach in writing health records?
- Is it OK to use accepted jargon and/or abbreviations in a health record?
- When should entries in a health record be made?
- Can I delete an entry, or alter part of an entry, in a health record that I made in error?
- Is it OK for me to ask a colleague to write entries in the patient's health record for me?
- Are there occasions when entries in a patient's health record have to be countersigned?
- Do I have to use black ink in a patient's health record?
- What constitutes good record keeping?
- Where and how should a health record be stored?
- How long do health records need to be kept before they can be destroyed?
- Can a patient read their own health record?
- How can a patient access their own health record?

(Continued)

- Can someone access their relative's health record?
- Can a parent or someone with parental responsibility access a child's health record?
- Can I, as a healthcare practitioner, access my own health record?
- Do the police have a right to see my patient's health record?
- What happens to health records after a patient's death?
- In summary, what strategy should a healthcare practitioner adopt when requested to disclose a patient's health record?

What is a health record?

Health record, medical record, treatment outcome, patient record, care summary, case notes, notes, integrated record, or any combination of these, are all used as terms for the collection of documents that relate to an individual's healthcare episode/s.

There are many ways to define what a health record is; if we turn to legislation to provide a definition, we could do worse than use the Data Protection Act 2018. It provides the following definition:

'Health record' means a record which

(a) consists of data concerning health, and

(b) has been made by or on behalf of a health professional in connection with the diagnosis, care or treatment of the individual to whom the data relates (Data Protection Act 2018: Section 205[1]).

From a legal perspective, a health record is anything that meets these criteria.

As to what a health record consists of, this can be as varied as the patients that you encounter. Some common elements will be featured in most health records whilst different groups of patients will have different items among their health records, with those within a specific group sharing common elements. As an example, if we consider a patient who is admitted to a medical assessment unit from the emergency department, we can trace some elements of their health record as they progress through their admission to discharge.

As the patient is admitted to the emergency department, they will have an admission sheet. Once they have been seen by the relevant healthcare practitioner, this may start to include an observation form; a history of the present complaint; a sheet detailing any allergies, their medication history and any current medication they are on; a prescription chart; blood investigations and results; other investigations and reports, for instance x-rays, electrocardiograms (ECGs); a diagnosis and treatment plan; a transfer summary for their admission to the medical assessment unit; healthcare practitioner notes for their time on the medical assessment unit; printouts from monitoring devices and equipment; a care plan; a form detailing their next of kin; notes made by any relevant specialist asked to advise on the patient's care and treatment; notes on clinical decision making. Once they are ready to be discharged, a discharge summary for their general practitioner (GP); outpatient medication record; any advice sheets for the patient; and details of any follow-up, including appropriate outpatient appointments.

We can all think of additional documents that could be added to this for individual specialities: photographs of an injury site or skin condition, notes from a consultation, video recording, consent forms, theatre operation forms, and so on. The longer the patient is under the care of the healthcare practitioner, the greater the number of documents that will comprise the patient's health record.

Essentially, a health record is anything and everything that refers to an identifiable individual patient and/or their care and treatment. To be classified as a 'health record', as opposed to any other form of record, the health record must contain information that has been recorded by or for a healthcare practitioner.

It is important to remember that health records which exist solely in an electronic format have the same ethical and legal principles, such as confidentiality, applied to them as paper-based health records, as they still meet the criteria for being a health record.

What is the purpose of a health record?

Just as we saw in the previous question that there are many ways of describing or naming a health record, so there are many ways in which a health record can be used. Health records are confidential documents and therefore there are only certain permitted ways in which they can be accessed and the information within them released. Not all of these uses will be discussed here but they can be categorised into three main purposes.

These three purposes for having health records are: 'clinical' and 'non-clinical', both of which benefit the patient, and 'other' where it doesn't necessarily. Examining these further the first, and some may say primary, purpose to a health record is clinical, ensuring that the patient receives the care and treatment they require. 'Clinical' refers to anything that is related to the healthcare experience and needs of the patient.

An individual health record should be a complete record of the patient's health history. As such, they provide an overview of the patient's health history; the patient's history of interactions with the healthcare system and healthcare practitioners, including previous clinical information, in relation to specific episodes of care and treatment that the patient has received; their current illness or condition; their current medication, and the care and/or treatment they are receiving; as well as providing planning for their future care and treatment needs. Information about clinical decision making should also be included. 'Clinical' also refers to the information collected about the patient, their name, date of birth, relationships, allergies, religious beliefs, and so on during these episodes of healthcare and treatment.

Health records are a way in which members of the patient's multidisciplinary healthcare team can communicate with each other about the patient and their plans for the care and treatment. No healthcare practitioner is available 24 hours a day during a patient's health episode. Therefore, a healthcare practitioner needs to ensure that other healthcare practitioners are aware of their interactions with the patient and any plans they have put in place regarding the patient's care and treatment.

'Non-clinical' refers to anything that is related to the patient but is not a clinical need, for instance if the patient was applying for a job and information was requested from the prospective employer's occupational health department regarding whether the patient was fit to undertake the duties of the job. In this example, the health record could be reviewed to provide the basis for a reply to the occupational health department.

'Other' refers to things that are not directly for the benefit of the patient, for instance resource management, audit purposes, quality assurance. Patient health records can be used as part of a research study collecting anonymised data on the outcome of certain types of accident; or to determine the frequency of certain types of treatment in order to provide adequate healthcare provision in a given area; or to demonstrate that staffing levels are adequate or not; or in the collection of legally required data such as the statutory requirement for statistical data to be kept in relation to certain procedures, for instance abortion and infertility treatments.

Where the patient's health record is being used for research, audit, statistical, or reporting purposes, whenever possible the information being used, for instance to complete a report, should be anonymised.

There is an old saying that goes something like: if you didn't write it down, it didn't happen. I have heard this most often in relation to healthcare practitioners and their records. If you or another healthcare practitioner from your healthcare team ever faces a disciplinary, regulatory body or legal case relating to your clinical practice, your patient's health records will most likely be examined. The old saying will come into play and, if you cannot rely on your record keeping to show that something happened the way you say it did, you may find that others may assume it did not happen the way you say. In a court case, the patient record is the strongest evidence; if something is missing, it will then be the patient's memory and recollection of events that is considered, only after this will your recollection be used. In short, if you don't record it in the patient's health record, there will be no evidence to support you and your actions.

Health records allow for information to be recorded and to not have to rely on the memory of the healthcare practitioner. Health records allow for information to be passed to and from the members of the multidisciplinary healthcare team. They provide for continuity of care and treatment, even when some members of the healthcare team are not present. Health records also provide evidence that procedures and treatment have been performed.

Some healthcare practitioners, such as general practitioners and midwives, are required by law to keep a record of certain types of interaction with their patients, and the health record meets this legal requirement.

It is often said that health records are 'legal documents' and, as such, can be used in a court of law. The fact is that a court can order the production of any document relating to a case before it, and this could include the whole of a health record or any specific document relating to the care and/or treatment of a particular patient.

Q

Who owns and controls a health record?

A

Many individuals, including patients themselves, believe that as the information in a health record concerns one individual, that individual, the patient, owns and is able to control what happens to a health record. As we shall see, this is not the case.

For patients who are treated within the National Health Service (NHS), health records are owned in the name of the Secretary of State for Health. In practice, the NHS Trust who provided the treatment for the patient are considered the owner of health records. If the patient has been treated privately but on behalf of the NHS, then the records will still be under the ownership of the Secretary of State for Health.

If the healthcare practitioner works for an employer outside of the NHS, generally it will be that employer who owns the health record and documentation that is produced by healthcare practitioners employed by them. This is generally noted in the healthcare practitioner's contract of employment. However, as this is a general principle, healthcare practitioners should check with their employers as to ownership and control arrangements regarding health records and documentation.

For healthcare practitioners who undertake voluntary work, it can be uncertain whether it is the voluntary organisation or the healthcare practitioner who own any health record and documentation produced by the healthcare practitioner. If you find yourself in such a situation you would be best advised to clarify with the voluntary organisation who owns and controls the health record. Also, if it is not you that owns the health record, that you're able to gain access to those records for your own purposes when you need to, for instance if you were to face any regulatory or legal inquiry into your practice.

If you work in a private capacity, that is you are self-employed or otherwise do not have an employing organisation, it is most likely that you will be the owner of the health records and documentation that you produce in the course of your clinical practice. If this is the case, then you should seek professional advice regarding their storage, retention and eventual disposal arrangements.

Just because someone owns and is therefore able to control a health record this does not mean that they are able to do as they wish with the health record. Health records are subject to the principles of confidentiality discussed in the previous chapter and it is the owner of the health record that is liable for their safekeeping, and for their eventual destruction in accordance with any regulations in place at the relevant time.

What problems can arise with a health record?

The reason that health records can be problematic is because they are poorly written or kept. There are two main issues which arise from a poor patient health record. The first is that it can result in issues for the patient and the second is that it can cause issues and/or implications for the healthcare practitioner(s).

With regard to the patient, poor record keeping can undermine and compromise the care and/or treatment they are receiving or even result in their harm. As I have previously noted, this is because:

> as one of the functions of a health care record is to provide a means for communication regarding a patient's health events, poor record keeping can hamper that communication: both with the patient and with other members of the health care team.

> If tests that are ordered are not recorded, or the results not entered into the patient's health care record, tests may be repeated. This is wasteful in terms of time and resources as well as potentially harmful to the patient.

> If the health care record is incomplete in terms of the patient's past health history, the patient's details regarding a specific condition may be missing, the patient's response to certain treatment may be lacking, previous symptoms and response to treatment may be imprecise. All of which may result in a delayed diagnosis or inappropriate treatment being given.

> And, as a consequence of the above, patients may lose confidence in the ability of the health care practitioners looking after them (Cornock, 2019: 35–6).

With regards to healthcare practitioners, the consequences of poor record keeping can mean that the healthcare practitioner is more susceptible to disciplinary and/or legal and/or healthcare regulatory body fitness to practise investigations. If such an investigation(s) were to occur, the healthcare practitioner may find that, if their record keeping is poor, they are unable to substantiate the care and treatment they have provided. In a court of law, if there is no record, such as an entry in a patient's health record, that an event took place, the court will infer that it did not happen, and this will hamper any defence put forward on their behalf as the opposing side will receive the benefit of the doubt. Also, if your record keeping is found to be below the acceptable standard, this may raise doubts about other aspects of your practice.

For the healthcare practitioner, poor record keeping by them can lead to their clinical practice being questioned, their employment being in jeopardy, the possibility of a legal case being brought against them, as well as their registration being put at risk.

There are many ways in which record keeping can be considered to be 'poor' or below the accepted standard; examples include:

- not having a single record for a patient but notes across different sets of records
- health records that are disorganised or difficult to navigate meaning that it is difficult to find information or specific entries
- information put in inappropriate parts of the health record, for instance future treatment plans being placed in with previous admissions
- the use of abbreviations that no-one understands
- health records that are not up to date
- incomplete entries, for instance, if a patient is reported as being in pain, what care or treatment was the patient given to alleviate the pain and did this work or not?
- incomplete health records with missing pages
- essential detail lacking, for instance, patient details, contact details for relatives, details regarding patient diagnosis or treatment, or review dates
- illegible entries
- no patient details on each page of entries so that it is not possible to state with absolute certainty that all the pages relate to the same patient
- phrases and terminology used inappropriately so that meaning is lost
- entries not signed or with an illegible signature, so it is not known who has written the entry
- health records that contain documents relating to two or more patients in a single patient record
- judgemental terms used in entries that are not substantiated, possibly leading to that entry and subsequent entries by the same healthcare practitioner to seem inaccurate and/or unprofessional
- an addition made but not indicated as such
- vague statements made in entries such as 'patient fine', 'no change', 'care given as requested' or 'slept well', meaning that it is not possible to know what care was given
- non-chronological entries, meaning it is not possible to follow the patient's progress
- entries obliterated but not obviously corrected
- dates, times, signatures, and so on missing from entries.

Q Is there a standard, either legal or regulatory, I have to reach in writing health records?

A There is no specific standard, either legal or from one of the healthcare regulatory bodies, which states the exact way in which a healthcare practitioner has to write the health records for the patients; although there are general principles which exist to guide the healthcare practitioner in their writing of health records. For instance, both the Health and Care Professions Council and the Nursing and Midwifery Council have statements in their respective codes of conduct in relation to the keeping of health records.

The Health and Care Professions Council's code of conduct states:

Keep accurate records

10.1 You must keep full, clear, and accurate records for everyone you care for, treat, or provide other services to.

10.2 You must complete all records promptly and as soon as possible after providing care, treatment or other services.

Keep records secure

10.3 You must keep records secure by protecting them from loss, damage or inappropriate access (Health and Care Professions Council, 2016: 10).

Whilst the Nursing and Midwifery Council's code states:

Keep clear and accurate records relevant to your practice.

This applies to the records that are relevant to your scope of practice. It includes but is not limited to patient records.

To achieve this, you must:

10.1 complete records at the time or as soon as possible after an event, recording if the notes are written some time after the event

10.2 identify any risks or problems that have arisen and the steps taken to deal with them, so that colleagues who use the records have all the information they need

10.3 complete records accurately and without any falsification, taking immediate and appropriate action if you become aware that someone has not kept to these requirements

10.4 attribute any entries you make in any paper or electronic records to yourself, making sure they are clearly written, dated and timed, and do not include unnecessary abbreviations, jargon or speculation

10.5 take all steps to make sure that records are kept securely

10.6 collect, treat and store all data and research findings appropriately (Nursing and Midwifery Council, 2018: 11).

What you can see from these extracts is that they are very general in what they expect from their respective registrants, although they do provide some general guidance relating to making sure that the health record is accurate and written as contemporaneously as possible.

Legally, the required standard for writing health records is the same as we met when considering **What is the legal standard I have to reach in my practice? (p. 46)**. This is the 'Bolam test' as modified by the 'Bolitho test'.

You may recall that the 'Bolam test' is that a healthcare practitioner must reach the standard of the ordinary competent practitioner professing to have the skills and knowledge required to undertake the specific action performed, and this standard must be capable of withstanding logical scrutiny.

Applying the 'Bolam test' to writing health records, a healthcare practitioner must ensure that in writing their health records they do so in a similar way to that of other healthcare practitioners, and that they can provide a rationale as to how and why they've written their health records in the way they have.

It is important to remember that your standard of care and practice will be judged by the standard of your record keeping. Poor record keeping may suggest to the reader that your standard of care is poor as well. As noted in **What problems can arise with a health record? (p. 134)**, it is not possible to provide an effective defence against allegations of poor practice or a complaint where a health record is inadequately written or is incomplete. Further, courts of law tend to draw adverse inferences from poor record keeping and where something is not documented will assume that it was not done.

Although there is no set standard for record keeping, and there are clear differences between the record keeping of individual healthcare practitioners, it is important to ensure that your record keeping is at least as good as your peers.

Is it OK to use accepted jargon and/or abbreviations in a health record?

You may have noticed that part of the Nursing and Midwifery Council's code stated, 'do not include unnecessary abbreviations, [or] jargon' (2018: 11). Does this mean that it is not acceptable to use jargon and/or abbreviations in health records?

There is no legal reason why jargon or abbreviations cannot be used in a patient's health record. As we have seen in **Is there a standard, either legal or regulatory, I have to reach in writing health records? (p. 135)** the healthcare regulatory bodies do not explicitly restrict their use either.

Although the use of jargon and abbreviations is not explicitly restricted, this does not mean that healthcare practitioners should use them indiscriminately or continuously throughout their writing in patient health records.

It must be possible for a health record to be read and understood by all the other healthcare practitioners who have to use it. If a healthcare practitioner is either not able to understand what is written or is unsure of what is meant by an entry, this defeats the point of having made the entry in the first place.

In using jargon and abbreviations, a healthcare practitioner should be mindful of why they are using it and what they are gaining by using it as opposed to writing in full prose. Some general points can be made regarding the use of jargon and abbreviations:

- keep the use of jargon and abbreviations to a minimum
- consider whether the jargon or abbreviations you are using is something that can be understood by all healthcare practitioners

- on first using an abbreviation, also write it out in full
- it is useful to have a list of abbreviations at the front or back of a particular health record
- use jargon in context, so that the potential for misunderstanding is reduced
- just because a particular term or abbreviation is in use in your hospital or clinic does not mean that it will be understood by other healthcare practitioners, so where possible, avoid the use of jargon, abbreviations and technical terms.

Q

When should entries in a health record be made?

A

When we considered **Is there a standard, either legal or regulatory, I have to reach in writing health records? (p. 135)** both the Health and Care Professions Council and the Nursing and Midwifery Council codes of conduct referred to completing records promptly and as soon as possible after the event. There are sound reasons for the healthcare regulatory bodies to consider it important enough that they include this in their respective codes of conduct.

I have previously noted that:

> as a health care record is a means of communication regarding a patient and their health event to the whole health care team, it is important that anyone coming into contact with the patient has the correct and up-to-date information available to them. The sooner a health care record is updated the sooner other members of the health care team will have access to the relevant information for their aspect of the patient's care and treatment.

> If a record is updated contemporaneously with the events it portrays, the less likely it is that investigations and their results will be overlooked and that referrals and follow up requirements will be missed.

> It can be argued that recording an event contemporaneously saves time as it means that the health care practitioner will not have to keep referring to their notes or refreshing their memory to record the event.

> Making a record at the time of the event means that it is more likely to be done and not forgotten. Delays in recording the event, making errors in the recording due to forgetting important details or making an inadequate record of the event can all lead to harm for the patient (Cornock, 2019: 36).

There are many reasons why health records are not updated during a healthcare practitioner's shift or after each patient encounter. Some overriding reasons may be a lack of time during the healthcare practitioner's shift and that not enough priority is given to recording care, the priority being to provide the care rather than record that it has been done.

Although we can sympathise with these reasons, if entries in health records are not made contemporaneously, there may be an issue regarding entries that are made retrospectively and particularly those that are made some time after the event being written about. The issue is related to the ability of an individual healthcare practitioner to fully remember all the details that need to be recorded in the health notes of a specific patient for a specific care episode. This is compounded when the healthcare practitioner has more than one patient that they have to make notes about. The question that needs to be asked is, how long after a care episode can a healthcare practitioner make an entry in a health record and still record all the relevant facts and detail? This will obviously vary between healthcare practitioners and most would not intentionally leave their record keeping to a time when they have forgotten pertinent details.

Yet, emergencies and other incidents can happen that take the healthcare practitioner away from the time they had allocated to record keeping, meaning that missing entries can be seen in patient health records.

As important as providing care and treatment to patients is, the healthcare practitioner also has a duty to ensure that they record these episodes for the benefit of the patient. Making entries as soon as possible after the relevant patient episode has occurred will help ensure that it is as accurate and complete as it can be, as it will be fresh in the healthcare practitioner's mind, and also, that the entry is actually made. This, in turn, will ensure that all members of the patient's multidisciplinary team are kept up to date regarding the patient's condition and that aspects of the patient's care are not delayed or overlooked.

 Can I delete an entry, or alter part of an entry, in a health record that I made in error?

 We all make mistakes. Some of the mistakes we make have more serious consequences than others. What is important, in the context of health records, is to know when we have made a mistake and to rectify that mistake clearly.

There is no legal, ethical or regulatory objection to the correction of an entry or part of an entry in a patient health record. In fact, where an entry is erroneous, correcting is to be welcomed. What is important is the way that the correction is undertaken.

If you are ever considering altering an entry in a health record without clearly indicating that this is a revision of a previous entry, one word of advice – *don't*. You would be surprised at what forensic document investigators can uncover. They have techniques that can determine if parts of an entry were written in different ink or at a different time to other parts, even when this is not visible to the naked eye. Other techniques can determine if the same person wrote the whole of an entry or if it was written by different individuals, so if someone were to change a previous entry made by another healthcare practitioner, this will be identified. With regard to electronic health records, the forensic investigator can determine the exact time that an entry was made, the computer it was made on, and the login details of the person making it, as well as when entries have been changed, overwritten or even deleted. Deleted entries can be recovered from health records even though an individual has taken steps to remove them.

Ideally, if an entry is noted to be erroneous in some way, it would be corrected by the healthcare practitioner who originally made it. In a paper-based health record, the entry to be corrected should be struck through with a single pen stroke so that it is still readable. The new entry should be put as close as possible to the one being corrected. Both entries should be dated and signed. A note should also be made as to the reason why the entry was erroneous.

If the entry is in an electronic health record, there are two possible ways of correcting an entry. Some systems will allow an entry to be identified as an error and a new entry to be written alongside, together with the reasons for the amendment. In systems where this is not possible, a new entry should be made, clearly identifying the entry that needs to be amended, along with the incorrect information, and the amended entry should then immediately follow this.

Where it is not possible for the erroneous entry to be corrected by the person who originally made it, another healthcare practitioner may correct the entry but in doing so should note that they are making the correction on behalf of the original healthcare practitioner and why.

Regardless of whoever amends an incorrect entry or whether it is done on a paper or electronic-based system, both the original entry and the revised entry need to be clearly identified and readable.

Q **Is it OK for me to ask a colleague to write entries in the patient's health record for me?**

A Healthcare practitioners are accountable to their patients and their colleagues to ensure that they record their interactions with their patients, as well as the results of any investigations they perform, any diagnosis they reach, and any care and treatment plans they formulate, in the patient's health record.

The entry you make in a patient's health record can be used as evidence of your interactions with your patient as well as demonstrating that you have fulfilled your duty of care to them, by providing a detailed account of the care and treatment you have provided and have planned for the patient. If someone else were to write the entry in the patient's health record it could be taken to mean that you have not fulfilled your duty to the patient yourself.

Asking another healthcare practitioner to make entries in the patient's health record on your behalf is not something to be advised. It is certainly not something that should be undertaken as a matter of routine or regularly. How do you know that they will do it correctly?

If someone were to ask you to write their entry in their patient's health record for them your best course of action would be to refuse. If you were to make the entry you would be doing so using someone else's information that they have passed on to you. You would be interpreting their information to make the entry. You need to question whether this is best for the patient and their clinical needs. How would you feel if you made an error in the entry? Could your actions in making an entry for someone else cause harm to the patient?

Every healthcare practitioner should make their own entries, unless there is an overwhelming reason why this cannot be done. Where it absolutely has to be made by another healthcare practitioner, that person should explicitly indicate that they are making the entry on behalf of someone else, naming that person and their role, make the entry and sign it themselves, clearly indicating their role as well. They should note the time of any interactions by the other healthcare practitioner with the patient, as well as the time they are making the entry. They should also note any information given to them by the healthcare practitioner, asking them to make the entry.

Where an entry in a patient's health record has been made by someone other than the healthcare practitioner providing the specific care and treatment being recorded, both healthcare practitioners, the healthcare practitioner delegating the writing of the entry and the healthcare practitioner writing it, will be liable for its accuracy.

There is another point that should be made about colleagues and patient health records. This is about what to do when two or more healthcare practitioners disagree about a patient's care and/or treatment. Whilst this may not be a common occurrence, where it happens, both or all the healthcare practitioners should write an entry in the patient's health record that details their interpretation of the patient's condition and needs, and their proposed solution. Each should include the date and time and the entries should be signed by the respective healthcare practitioners, noting their role in the patient's multidisciplinary healthcare team.

 Are there occasions when entries in a patient's health record have to be countersigned?

The main occasion when an entry in a patient's health record should be countersigned is where the person making the entry is acting under the authority of someone else. For instance, where a healthcare practitioner has delegated the care of a patient to a student healthcare practitioner or someone not registered with one of the healthcare regulatory bodies. In this instance the person to whom the care has been delegated, such as the student nurse, may write the entry but this should be countersigned by the person who delegated the care, the registered nurse, as both individuals have liability in relation to the care delivered and the recording of that care.

Individual employers may have a policy in place regarding the writing of entries in patient health records by those who have a patient's care, or aspects of it, delegated to them. You should ensure that you follow any policy or guidance that exists. Where none exists, the comments above may be considered good practice.

When considering **Is it OK for me to ask a colleague to write entries in the patient's health record for me? (p. 140)**, it was noted that the healthcare practitioner making the entry should clearly indicate that they were making the entry of behalf of someone else, name them and state why they were doing so. It would be good practice for the healthcare practitioner who asked for the entry to be made to countersign the entry to confirm that it is an accurate reflection of the event being recorded. As noted, both healthcare practitioners would have liability for its accuracy, so both should indicate that they agree with its contents by signing the record.

Q Do I have to use black ink in a patient's health record?

A Your clinical area may have a policy or procedure that you will need to follow with regard to the specifics of completing an entry in a patient's health record. If there is no specific policy or procedure in place, you may follow these general principles.

There is no legal requirement to write a health record in a specific colour ink. What is required is that the entry is written legibly in an ink that is permanent. Black ink is sometimes said to be the preferred ink colour to use because it does not rub out without trace and is a colour that can be photocopied. Blue ink has similar properties. Ink colour can be an issue when entries are written in red or green, or especially if pencil were to be used in making entries in a patient's health record. For red and green ink, this is because they do not always photocopy well on black and white photocopiers, but they are generally OK on colour photocopiers, although this costs considerably more per page. Pencil is never recommended as a medium for writing in a patient's health record because it can easily be erased, and it does not photocopy well. Hence entries can be erased without your knowledge and/or may not show up on copies of health records.

Other things to consider in the actual writing of entries in a patient's health record are to not leave sections blank but to initial or put 'NA' in every box or section to indicate that you have noted the box or section but have nothing to enter in that area. Similarly, put a line through any blank pages or areas between the last entry and the one you are making. This will prevent anyone inadvertently putting an entry before your entry and so confusing the chronology of the health record. If there are any loose pages, either fix these into the record or staple them to a page of the health record and note what you have done.

Q What constitutes good record keeping?

A Good record keeping is record keeping that results in an effective health record for the patient. To be effective, a health record needs to provide members of the multidisciplinary healthcare team with the information they need to fulfil their role in the team and provide the best possible healthcare to the patient.

A good health record is one that can be picked up by any healthcare practitioner and they will be able to determine the episodes of healthcare that the patient has had and, for each of those episodes, they can reconstruct from the records the details of the episode and if/how it affects the patient's current health needs. This is because good record keeping allows the patient's health timeline to be established as well as the timeframe for each individual health episode, as well as containing accurate, factual and comprehensive information.

There are always going to be calls on the time of the healthcare practitioner that can take them away from their record keeping. Maintaining good record keeping does not mean that a healthcare practitioner needs to spend more time on the writing of the health record than they do on the actual care and treatment provided to the patient. It does however mean that they need to adopt behaviours and techniques that become a routine so that the healthcare practitioner maintains their records efficiently.

Some of the features of a good health record are that it:

- clearly identifies the patient on each page and individual document
- is chronological, so that there is a logical progression from one entry to another and overall, from past to present events
- is legible in terms of the actual writing as well as the content, which should accurately reflect the interaction that the healthcare practitioner has had with the patient, without being open to misinterpretation
- details the patient's history of their current illness/condition as well as findings on examination and results of investigations, and where a diagnosis is made, the diagnosis and any alternatives and the basis for making the diagnosis
- will describe the decision-making process, including any information provided to the patient and the patient's involvement in the decision-making process
- will include details of any admission, procedures undertaken, further investigations, follow-up appointments and/or referrals
- records details of the patient's progress and evaluates care and treatment given to the patient, noting any changes to the patient's care or treatment as a consequence of that evaluation
- states where advice or information is given to the patient and what advice was given, and any patient response
- is succinct and easy to read, so that it does not take too much time to absorb the relevant information
- is a permanent record and cannot be altered or corrected without it being obvious this has been done
- where an entry has been corrected, this is obvious to anyone reading the entry and any amended entry is placed as near to the corrected entry as possible
- uses standard terminology, and explains all terms and abbreviations used that are not in common usage
- is written contemporaneously and, where a delay has occurred, the reason for the delay is stated
- identifies who wrote each entry
- has a list of signatures and who the corresponding person is
- has each document clearly dated, including the year, and each entry is timed using the 24-hour clock so there is no confusion as to whether an entry is AM or PM

- is complete
- is meaningful both to the healthcare practitioner who wrote it and the person who reads it.

Good record keeping is a hallmark of the highest standard of practice by healthcare practitioners; it demonstrates the highest standard of patient care. Where necessary, it allows a healthcare practitioner's practice to be defended years after the event occurred and where the healthcare practitioners involved may have changed jobs or roles or be otherwise uncontactable.

The key to good record keeping is to consider whether other members of the patient's multidisciplinary team are able to access all the information they need about your interactions with the patient when they cannot discuss them with you.

In summary, good record keeping results in patient health records that succinctly, accurately and chronologically presents factual information so that episodes relating to the patient's interaction with healthcare practitioners can be reconstructed solely from the information contained in the health record.

Where and how should a health record be stored?

As we noted in the chapter dealing with confidentiality, patients have an expectation that the information they provide to healthcare practitioners will remain confidential. If a health record is not stored in a way that will keep them secure, confidentiality may be breached. In addition, health records need to have their integrity maintained. This means that individual forms or sheets of paper are not detached from their patient folder and that computer records do not have corrupted or missing data.

It would be easy for all health records to be kept in a locked room and access restricted so that they can only be consulted in that room and never taken out. Whilst this would probably deal with the issue of confidentiality and keep the records secure, it would not be practical in terms of access to the health record by those who need the information it contains in order to treat and care for patients.

It is this balance between maintaining confidentiality and keeping the health record secure and ensuring that it is accessible to those who need it, but restricted from unauthorised individuals, that can pose problems in the storage of health records.

Logic states that to do this health records should not be left where unauthorised individuals can access them. For paper-based health records, this may mean keeping them in an area away from public access. If the health record is in an electronic format, this would mean ensuring that computers are protected from all unauthorised use, through systems such as a requirement for username and password entry, and that monitors displaying confidential information cannot be viewed by unauthorised individuals.

Where health records need to be carried by healthcare practitioners outside of a secure environment, for instance in making visits to patients' homes, extra care is needed to ensure that they are not left unattended or that electronic equipment is not left unsecured.

Healthcare practitioners should not remove health records from their area of employment, for instance taking them home so that they can complete their record keeping, without having express permission to do so.

Your employer will have guidance on the storage of health records and this needs to be followed. Failure to follow any guidance or policy that results in a health record being accessible by someone unauthorised could lead to disciplinary action by your employer and possibly a fitness to practise investigation by the relevant healthcare regulatory body.

Many healthcare practitioners make notes about the patients they are responsible for that they use during a specific shift or patient episode. These are often compiled during a handover from one healthcare practitioner to another. They usually contain basic information about a patient and their condition, and any specific items that the healthcare practitioner feels they need to care for or treat the patient. These need to be considered as part of the patient's health record until the information is transferred to the patient's permanent health record or it is no longer needed by the healthcare practitioner, when it should be securely destroyed in accordance with any local policies or guidance (but see section on clinical diaries in **How long do health records need to be kept before they can be destroyed? [p. 145]**).

Q

How long do health records need to be kept before they can be destroyed?

A

When discussing **What is a health record? (p. 130)**, we saw that most documents that relate to the care and treatment of a patient can be considered part of a health record and therefore need to be retained as part of an individual patient's health record. This means that for some patients their health records can be quite large and consist of many individual documents.

At some point in time, a decision will need to be made as to whether the documents within a health record, or the whole health record, should be destroyed. This may be because of the death of the patient, or because there has been no activity in relation to the health record for a number of years, or because individual documents within the health record are no longer considered to be clinically relevant.

It could be considered good practice to destroy documents relating to a specific episode of a patient's care and treatment once that episode has been concluded. This negates the risk of any confidentiality breach related to their storage. However, for many patient healthcare episodes, it is not known whether the illness or condition will return or if specific episodes will have relevance to any future healthcare episodes that the patient may experience. Additionally, there are reasons that necessitate health records to be retained even if they are not clinically required, such as statutory requirements. For all these reasons, detailed guidance has been developed regarding the retention and destruction of health records.

For those healthcare practitioners working in the National Health Service (NHS), the current guidance relating to the management of health records is the *Records Management Code of Practice for Health and Social Care 2016* (Information Governance Alliance, 2016). This is a very detailed document that provides guidance not only in relation to the minimum period that health records need to be retained and how they should be destroyed, but also in relation to their storage, including the design of storage systems.

For a healthcare practitioner working outside of the NHS, their employer's policies should be consulted for guidance relating to the retention and destruction of health records. For self-employed healthcare practitioners, advice can be sought from professional organisations or legal advisers regarding retention and destruction of records. However, the NHS guidance can be considered to represent best practice.

In general, the guidance is that health records should be retained for a minimum period of eight years after the patient was last seen, the conclusion of a specific period of treatment, or their death. However, if the health record relates to a child, it should be retained to at least the patient's 25th birthday or 26th birthday if they were 17 when their treatment was concluded.

These minimum periods of retention increase for specific types of record and for records relating to specific healthcare specialities. For instance, general practitioner (GP) records must be kept for a minimum of 10 years after the patient's death; mental health records made in relation to a patient who has been cared for or treated under the provisions of the Mental Health Act 1983 for a minimum of 20 years, or eight years after the death of the patient; obstetric records for a minimum of 25 years; and records in relation to patients receiving oncology diagnosis and/or treatment for a minimum of 30 years, or eight years after the death of the patient. Where the health record relates to a long-term illness that has the potential to recur, or is a lifelong illness, the minimum retention period increases to 30 years, or eight years after the death of the patient.

CLINICAL DIARIES

Healthcare practitioners who use a diary to record details of their visits to patients and clients or to record details of clinical activity they have undertaken need to transfer this information to the patient's main health record. The clinical diary then needs to be kept for a minimum of two years from the end of that calendar year. Where the healthcare practitioner does not or cannot transfer the information to the patient's main health record, the clinical diary needs to be retained for a minimum of eight years from the end of the calendar year it relates to.

DESTRUCTION OF RECORDS

Prior to destruction, all health records need to be reviewed to see if there are any reasons that justify their continued retention as the retention periods in the guidance are a minimum rather than a maximum. If there is a reason to keep the health record or part of it for longer than the minimum period, for instance it relates to an obstetric episode, it must be retained and reviewed again at the end of the new retention period.

Once the minimum retention period has expired, and assuming there are no more reasons to justify the retention of the health record, the health record must be destroyed according to any policy in place at the time but, as a minimum, destruction must occur in such a way that information cannot be retrieved.

Can a patient read their own health record?

When we considered **Who owns and controls a health record? (p. 133)** we saw that health records are not owned by the people they are about.

If you own a set of documents, you can control what happens to them and this would include reading them yourself. When you don't own the documents, this access is not automatic but one that you must request. This is the situation that patients legally find themselves in when they want to read their own health records. They do not own the records and therefore cannot access them or read them without requesting permission.

The problem with this is that patients can sometimes freely access their health record or parts of it when they are receiving care and treatment in hospital or clinics. This is because health records can be left unattended at the end of a patient's bed or otherwise unattended where they are not supervised. In either case, whilst most patients may not look at their own health record, some may.

If a patient is seen to be reading their own health record, they need to be told that this is something that they should not be doing, and that they should ask if they have specific questions about their care or treatment, or if they want additional information from their health record, they should request access to it.

This does not prevent a healthcare practitioner from sharing an entry they have made or some test results, but this is at the healthcare practitioner's discretion and is not a patient's automatic right.

This question also raises another issue, that of the language used in writing an entry in a patient's health record. Although the patient has no automatic right to access and read their own health record, would they be able to understand the entry that you had made? If the entries are not written in language that the patient can understand, why not? Can you amend how you write your entries so that they could be understood by the patient they relate to? If the entry is written in language that the patient could understand, this will ensure that other healthcare practitioners can also understand it.

If, on the other hand, you would not want your patient to see the entry you have made in their health record, you need to reflect on why this is and consider if the way you undertake your record keeping meets what is expected from a healthcare practitioner. If it doesn't, you may need to change the way you write your records.

Q **How can a patient access their own health record?**

A Patients have several statutes on their side if they want to access their health records, depending upon their reason for wanting to see their health record.

If the patient is making a claim, or considering making a claim, against a healthcare practitioner, hospital or clinic for alleged negligence, the Supreme Court Act 1981 may provide access to their health record. Section 33(2) of this Act provides that, if a patient were to apply to the High Court, it may order someone to disclose what documents they have and to provide these documents to the applicant (the patient) or to the patient's representatives. The High Court has to be convinced that there is a real prospect of litigation commencing before they will order the release of the health record.

If the patient wanted to see a health record that was being prepared on them for employment or insurance purposes, the Access to Medical Reports Act 1988 provides the necessary authority. The right in the Act extends to seeing the report in the health record before it is sent to the prospective employer or insurer, as well as after it has been sent. As well as a right to see the report, the Act also gives the patient the right to stop the report being forwarded to the prospective employer or insurer and to request that the report is amended, if they consider that it is incorrect or misleading in any way, or to have a statement attached to the report if the healthcare practitioner will not alter the report (Section 5).

If the patient has died and their representatives want access to their health record, the Access to Health Records Act 1990 is relevant as Section 3 allows this where a claim may arise as a result of the patient's death. This Act was at one time the main statutory provision relating to access to health records but was superseded by the Data Protection Act 1998, apart from Section 3, as the Data Protection Act 1998 did not provide for access by the representatives of the deceased person's estate. The Access to Health Records Act 1990 covers health records created since 1st November 1991.

The Freedom of Information Act 2000 may be thought to be useful legislation in accessing a health record held by a public body, i.e. the National Health Service (NHS). However, health information is not covered in the provisions of the Act as it is personal information.

The above has shown how someone can access health records in specific circumstances. More generally, the main statutory provision which allows a patient to access their health record is the Data Protection Act 2018 (DPA), which replaced the Data Protection Act 1998, and allows the General Data Protection Regulation of the European Union to become law in the United Kingdom.

The DPA provides access to personal data that is being held about someone on request to the controller of that data. From a patient's perspective, personal data includes health records and so this is a means by which a patient can gain access to their health record. The Act requires a controller of data, who has received a subject access request (the term given to someone asking for their own personal data), to provide to that person details of the information that is held about them, along with details of how the information is being processed (used) and a copy of the information. Apart from exceptional circumstances, the controller cannot charge a fee for supplying the information and it has to be in a format that the subject can understand.

As well as requesting access to their health records, patients also have the right to ask for corrections to be made if there are inaccuracies present.

Although the DPA gives patients wide-ranging access to their health records, there are exemptions to this. The most common exemptions are:

- where the healthcare practitioner believes that disclosing the information would cause serious harm to the physical or mental health of the individual or another person
- where disclosing the information would also disclose information about a third person.

These exemptions apply not only to access under the DPA but to any of the ways, discussed above, that a patient can access their health record. If any aspect of the health record is withheld, this must be explained to the patient.

Before a patient is allowed access to their record, the record needs to be checked to ensure that third party confidentiality will not be breached and that there is no risk of serious harm to the patient or anyone else from the disclosure of the health record to the patient.

A patient may also make a request to a specific healthcare practitioner providing care or treatment to them for access to their health record. It is a judgement for the individual healthcare practitioner as to whether they share their part of the health record with the patient, after considering the two exemptions detailed above. However, they cannot share something that has not originated from them, for instance entries made by another healthcare practitioner, without that person's express permission. Healthcare practitioners should know their employer's or clinical area's policy on patients accessing their health records.

Can someone access their relative's health record?

As we saw in **How can information be shared without breaching confidentiality?** (**p. 108**), one way to legally and ethically share information is with the consent of the patient. This applies to health records as well.

It is important to reiterate that for a healthcare practitioner to be able to rely upon the patient's consent as justification for the release of their confidential information, that consent needs to be legally valid consent. When identifying **What criteria must be fulfilled for consent to be legally valid? (p. 68)**, it was noted that there are four legal principles which must be fulfilled for the consent given by the patient to be valid.

If the patient is willing to give their consent, their health record could be shared with their relatives if the healthcare practitioner considers it appropriate to do so. However, if the patient is unwilling to provide their consent, the health record cannot be shared with their relatives. The Data Protection Act 2018, which provides patients with the right to make a subject access request for their own health record, does not extend to someone requesting a health record on behalf of someone else.

Where the patient is not competent to make a decision regarding whether their health record should be shared with their relatives, the healthcare practitioner needs to consider whether it is in the best interests of the patient for it to be shared (see **How can information be shared without breaching confidentiality? [p. 108]**). It may be that information can be shared with relatives about the patient's condition, treatment and/or prognosis and so on without actually providing relatives with access to the patient's health record.

The Mental Capacity Act 2005 contains provisions for individuals to be identified to act on the patient's behalf when the patient is incompetent to do so. These are known as 'lasting powers of attorney' (see **Are there any circumstances in which someone can consent on behalf of an adult patient? [p. 86]**) and may entitle the nominated individual to gain access to parts of the patient's health record.

Even if it is considered in the best interests of the patient to share their health record with the relative, this does not mean that the relative or the nominated individual with a lasting power of attorney has free access to the whole of the patient's health record. Rather it means that specific parts of the health record relating to the patient's current condition may be shared in order that the relative may make decisions relating to the patient's care and treatment or make general decisions on the patient's behalf.

In the usual way, parts of the health record should be withheld if they refer to third parties or if they could cause serious mental or physical harm to the patient or others. If any aspect of the health record is withheld, this must be explained to the relatives.

Q Can a parent or someone with parental responsibility access a child's health record?

A In **Are children able to consent to their own treatment? (p. 82)** it was noted that from a legal perspective a child is anyone under the age of 18. Also, that a child over the age of 16 is considered, again from a legal perspective, to be competent to provide their own consent, whilst those under 16 have to demonstrate that they are competent to consent.

The same legal principles regarding consent apply to a child's ability to request access to their own health record. The Data Protection Act 2018 allows the child over 16 to make a subject access request and children under 16, who can demonstrate that they have a sufficient understanding of the issues involved, may also make a subject access request. It is the controller of the health record who needs to determine whether a child under 16 lacks the competence to make a subject access request before refusing to supply the information requested.

Parents or those with parental responsibility (see **Who is a parent and who has parental responsibility? [p. 180]**) may request access to their child's health record. The health record can be supplied to a parent or someone with parental responsibility either with the consent of the child or when the child is not considered competent to make decisions regarding their health records. Where only one parent has made a request for access, it is not necessary to inform the other parent or others with parental responsibility that access has been provided.

If a healthcare practitioner or other person in control of a health record considers that it is not in the child's best interests to give access to the parent, they may refuse access. Access may also be refused where it is considered that to provide access would cause serious harm to the child or to another person.

Where access is granted to someone with parental responsibility, access will be to the whole record unless it relates to a third party; that part will be withheld if consent cannot be obtained from the third party. If any part of the child's health record is withheld, this needs to be explained to the person being granted access.

Generally, where the child has the necessary competence to make decisions regarding access to their health records, providing access to a parent would only be done with the child's consent.

Can I, as a healthcare practitioner, access my own health record?

The same principles that apply to patients who want to read and access their health record apply to you. Being a healthcare practitioner does not give you any additional rights regarding accessing your own health record.

In some ways, you can be considered to be at more of a disadvantage than a patient who reads or accesses their own health record whilst in a hospital or otherwise receiving treatment, because you could be subject to disciplinary and/or healthcare regulatory body fitness to practise investigation for unauthorised access to your health record.

As a healthcare practitioner, you are only authorised to access health records for patients for whom you need access in order to provide care and treatment to them.

The same holds true if you were to access a friend's, relative's, neighbour's or colleague's health record even at their own request. In such circumstances, best practice would be to inform the person asking you to access their health record that you are unable to do so and to give them details of how they may access their health record themselves.

Do the police have a right to see my patient's health record?

The police do not have an automatic right to see a patient's health record. They may request access to a particular patient's health record but, unless access is given voluntarily, they will need to obtain a court order or a warrant.

To provide access to a patient's health record voluntarily, the healthcare practitioner either needs the consent of the patient, or they need to be acting in the public interest. Providing access to a health record in the public interest would include: the prevention, detection or prosecution of a serious crime, such as murder, rape or child abuse; threats to national security; terrorism; or where there is an identifiable threat to a third person.

Whilst the police have powers of investigation under the Police and Criminal Evidence Act 1984, personal records, such as health records, are deemed to be excluded material and as such the police are not usually able to demand access to them. If the police do require access to an individual's health record as part of their investigation into an offence, they can apply to the court for a special procedure warrant or court order from a judge.

Upon production of the court order or warrant, the healthcare practitioner is able to provide to the police the health record of the patient named on it. If the healthcare practitioner is in any doubt as to whether they can provide the police access to a patient's health record, they should seek appropriate guidance from their employer's legal department, a Caldicott Guardian, or their own legal representative such as from a trade union or indemnity provider.

Where access to a patient's health record is provided to the police, it should only be to the relevant parts of the health record.

What happens to health records after a patient's death?

After a patient's death, the duty of confidentiality owed by a healthcare practitioner continues to exist, although the provisions within the Data Protection Act 2018 no longer apply to the patient's health record. If there is a need to access the health records of a deceased patient, this can be via Section 3 of the Access to Health Records Act 1990, which covers health records created since 1st November 1991. Access is limited in terms of both the amount of access given to the health record and also in terms of those who can apply for access.

Access to a deceased patient's health record can be restricted for a number of reasons. Some of these reasons include:

- where the patient provided the information, the expectation that it would not be disclosed to others and/or the patient has included a note in their health record asking that the health record is not disclosed to a named individual

- where the information would identify a third party who has not consented to the release of their information, unless that third party is a healthcare practitioner who has provided care or treatment to the patient
- where a healthcare practitioner believes that releasing information in the health record could cause serious harm to the physical or mental health of a third party.

Those who can apply for access to the health record of a deceased patient include the patient's personal representatives and also those who may be able to make a claim on the deceased patient's estate. Those who request to access the health record will not automatically be given full access. Access is normally restricted to the information that is relevant to the access request.

There are statutory time limits within which access to health records must be provided, and the access must be provided free of charge.

Although the duty of confidentiality exists after the death of the patient, there are situations when the healthcare practitioner believes that disclosing information may either be something that the deceased patient would want or would be in the patient's best interests. For instance, the health record may contain information relating to genetic tests that the patient had had and there is a possibility that other members of the patient's family could be at risk of a hereditary disease. In a situation such as this, the healthcare practitioner may use their discretion in providing access to a limited aspect of the health record so that this information is available to those who may be at risk.

Death certificates, which form part of a patient's health record, are not confidential records. Further, coroners can ask for information contained in a deceased patient's health record in relation to an inquest.

Access to a deceased patient's health record is also legally permitted for the purposes of clinical audit and national confidential inquiries; and for public health reasons, although it should then be anonymised whenever possible.

 In summary, what strategy should a healthcare practitioner adopt when requested to disclose a patient's health record?

 In considering how to respond to a request for access to a patient's health record or for a disclosure to be made from the patient's health record, the healthcare practitioner should ask themselves several questions:

- Who is asking for the access or disclosure?
- What reason have they given?
- Is the patient alive or dead?
- If alive, is the patient competent to give their consent to the access or disclosure?
- If the patient is not competent to consent, or is dead, is there justification for access or disclosure to be made?

Once these questions have been answered, if the healthcare practitioner believes that access or disclosure may be justified, they should clearly identify their reason for giving access to that person, for example a subject access request from a competent patient or a request from a lawyer dealing with a patient's estate, and if necessary, take advice on their proposed course of action.

If access to the health record or disclosure is still justified, the healthcare practitioner should record any actions they have taken and who they have provided access to, or disclosed information to, and the extent of the disclosure.

SUMMARY

- Health records are important to record what care and treatment the patient has received, and what is planned.
- A health record is a set of documents relating to the health of an individual that has been made by, or on behalf of, a healthcare practitioner.
- Health records can be used clinically or non-clinically for the patient's benefit, or for other reasons not directly related to the patient such as the collection of statistical information.
- Health records are generally owned by a healthcare practitioner's employer, unless they are self-employed.
- Poor record keeping can lead to problems for the patient and/or the healthcare practitioner(s).
- There are no explicit standards for writing health records, although there are general principles that need to be followed.
- Whilst it is acceptable to use accepted abbreviations and jargon in a health record, this should be kept to an absolute minimum and their use should be explained.
- Entries in health records should be made as contemporaneously as possible.
- Correction of erroneous entries in a health record should be clear and allow other readers to identify the entry that is erroneous as well as the correction.
- Healthcare practitioners are accountable for ensuring that they record their own interactions with their patients as well as their patient's care and treatment plans.
- Entries made in a patient's health record do not normally have to be counter-signed unless care is delegated to another practitioner by someone retaining liability for that care when both should sign the entry.
- Ensure you write legibly and in permanent ink in a paper-based health record.
- Good record keeping provides members of the multidisciplinary healthcare team with the information they need to fulfil their role in the team in providing the best possible healthcare to the patient.
- Health records need to be stored so that the information within them remains confidential.

- There are specific time periods that health records, or parts of health records, need to be kept before they can be destroyed.
- Patients have no automatic right to read their health records or notes and need to request access if they wish to do so.
- There are various statutory provisions which allow a patient or their representatives to access their health record in certain circumstances. The main way that a person can gain access to their health record is via the provisions in the Data Protection Act 2018, although there are some exemptions which limit the release of health records.
- Relatives have no automatic right of access to a patient's health record. Specific parts of an incompetent patient's health record may be shared with relatives in the patient's best interests or when an individual has a Lasting Power of Attorney in relation to the patient.
- A competent child is entitled to request access to their own health record, and parents and those with parental responsibility may request access either with the consent of the child or on behalf of a child lacking competence.
- As a healthcare practitioner, you have no more right to access your health record than any other individual.
- The police may request access to a patient's health record and access may be given voluntarily by the healthcare practitioner or because the police have a court order or warrant granting them access.
- Health records remain confidential after the death of the patient, although access is permitted under the Access to Health Records Act 1990 for personal representatives and those with a legitimate reason to access the health record.

REFERENCES

Access to Health Records Act 1990.
Access to Medical Reports Act 1988.
Cornock, M. (2019) 'Record keeping and documentation: a legal perspective', *Orthopaedic and Trauma Times*, 35: 34–8.
Data Protection Act 1998.
Data Protection Act 2018.
Freedom of Information Act 2000.
General Data Protection Regulation 2016/679/EU.
Health and Care Professions Council (2016) *Standards of conduct, performance and ethics*. Health and Care Professions Council: London.
Information Governance Alliance (2016) *Records Management Code of Practice for Health and Social Care 2016*. Information Governance Alliance: London.
Mental Capacity Act 2005.
Mental Health Act 1983.
Nursing and Midwifery Council (2018) *The Code*. Nursing and Midwifery Council: London.
Police and Criminal Evidence Act 1984.
Supreme Court Act 1981.

DRUGS AND PRESCRIBING

This chapter considers how healthcare practitioners interact with drugs/medications from a legal and ethical perspective. This includes how a healthcare practitioner may prescribe drugs to patients and how they may manage a patient's drugs in clinical settings.

In this chapter, the word 'drug(s)' is being used as shorthand to mean medication prescribed for patients, unless specifically stated otherwise.

QUESTIONS COVERED IN CHAPTER 7

- What is a drug?
- How are drugs classified?
- What is a controlled drug?
- Is there a difference between prescribing and administering drugs?
- Do drugs have to be destroyed in certain ways?
- Can patients self-administer their drugs in a clinical setting?
- Is it ever appropriate to give a patient their drugs covertly?
- Can I use drugs from the ward drugs cupboard for my personal use?
- What should I do if asked by a senior healthcare practitioner to administer a drug that is not included in my employer's protocols?
- If possession of a controlled drug is unlawful, am I able to transport them to a patient in the community?
- What limits a healthcare practitioner's ability to prescribe drugs?
- Which healthcare practitioner groups can prescribe?
- What types of prescriber are there?
- As an independent prescriber, is it OK for me to prescribe drugs for my family members?
- As a non-prescriber, what can I do in relation to the prescribing of drugs to patients?
- What is a Patient Group Direction and is it a form of prescribing?
- Is there an agreed prescribing standard?

Q What is a drug?

A There are many definitions of 'drug' available should you choose to look for them, ranging from something that has medicinal properties, to compounds used in the practice of medicine, to illicit substances that can lead to addiction. All share a common element that can be used to describe a drug: this is that a drug is something that has a physical or psychological effect on the human body, generally used for diagnosing, treating or preventing disease, illness or a physical or psychological condition. In Acts and other legal contexts, drugs are usually referred to as medicinal products.

For a legal definition, we can turn to the Human Medicines Regulations 2012 where Section 2(1) provides that:

'medicinal product' means –

(a) any substance or combination of substances presented as having properties of preventing or treating disease in human beings; or

(b) any substance or combination of substances that may be used by or administered to human beings with a view to –

    (i) restoring, correcting or modifying a physiological function by exerting a pharmacological, immunological or metabolic action, or

    (ii) making a medical diagnosis.

Q How are drugs classified?

A The Medicines Act 1968 was a major development in the licensing of drugs in the United Kingdom. It has been repealed in part in recent years, most notably by the Human Medicines Regulations 2012. One of the features of the original Act was that it categorised drugs into three classes. These classes are:

- General Sale List (GSL) medicines
- Pharmacy (P) medicines
- Prescription only medicines (POM).

Different characteristics apply to drugs dependent upon in which class they are placed.

A drug on the GSL are also known as 'over the counter' or OTC drugs and may be sold and supplied without the presence of a pharmacist in places such as supermarkets. Paracetamol is an example of a drug on the GSL.

P medicines are those drugs that have a form of control in their supply, in that they can only be sold and supplied from a retail pharmacy business, a registered pharmacy or where the supply can be supervised by a pharmacist. An example of pharmacy medicines is the morning after pill.

POMs are drugs that can only be supplied under the guidance of an authorised healthcare practitioner through the writing of a prescription, which will detail the drug and dose to be supplied. An example of a POM is oral antibiotics.

As can be seen, the three classes of drug are a hierarchy moving from GSL through P to POM, with the restrictions on sale and supply being more onerous and restrictive as one moves through the list.

Q **What is a controlled drug?**

A In addition to the three classifications of drugs identified in **How are drugs classified? (p. 157)**, there is a further category of drugs whose properties mean that their supply needs to be controlled further than is possible as a prescription only medicine (POM). These are known as 'controlled drugs'. The reason for the further control is due to the potential for misuse that these drugs present.

A controlled drug is controlled in the sense that: its import and export is controlled; its manufacture is controlled; its supply is controlled; its possession is controlled; and, certain other activities in relation to the drug are limited, such as how it is used. Failure to follow the control measures is a criminal offence.

As an example, penicillin is POM. This means that you cannot obtain it without a prescription. Once it has been dispensed, the restriction on it is satisfied so that, if it was prescribed to my family member, I would be allowed to have it in my possession even if my family member was not present. However, with a controlled drug, if I have it in my possession without a lawful reason for doing so, something that will satisfy the terms of the control on the drug such as having it to supply to a patient, I will be committing a criminal offence. I could be arrested, charged and, on conviction, may face a custodial sentence.

To be classified as a controlled drug, the drug must be listed in Schedule 2 of the Misuse of Drugs Act 1971. Schedule 2 has three subdivisions known as Parts 1, 2 and 3, which further classify controlled drugs as Class A, Class B and Class C drugs. The reason for the division of controlled drugs in A, B and C is to determine the potential criminal offence and the penalties that can be applied. Schedule 2 is a living list and drugs on it may move between the classifications or be removed, whilst others could be added. The earlier in the alphabet the controlled drug is classified, the higher the offence that is committed by breaching the control on the drug and the higher the potential criminal penalty.

The Misuse of Drugs Regulations 2001 also classifies controlled drugs for the restriction of their production, supply, possession and prescription. The reason for this is that the Misuse of Drugs Act 1971 is an umbrella Act, which means that it provides the overarching framework in relation to the misuse of drugs and for controlling drugs that have the potential to be abused. The Misuse of Drugs Regulations 2001 provides exemptions to the provisions of the Misuse of Drugs Act 1971 in certain stated circumstances and these exemptions are based upon the classification that the controlled drug is assigned.

The Misuse of Drugs Act 1971 essentially makes everything to do with controlled drugs unlawful whilst the various regulations, such as The Misuse of Drugs Regulations 2001, allow certain activities such as prescription, supply and administration of specified drugs to be permitted under stated circumstances.

The Misuse of Drugs Regulations 2001 classification is based on five schedules, numbered 1 to 5, of which Schedule 4 has two parts. Schedule 1 is related to drugs not normally used medicinally. The lower the schedule number, the more restrictions placed on the drug.

The following table (Table 7.1) has examples of the classification of controlled drugs.

Table 7.1 Examples of the classification of controlled drugs

Drug	Misuse of Drugs Act 1971 classification	The Misuse of Drugs Regulations 2001 classification
Morphine	A	2
Codeine	B	2
Diazepam	C	4 Part 1

Is there a difference between prescribing and administering drugs?

There are actually three main activities that need to be considered in relation to drugs in a clinical setting. These are prescribing, supplying and administering drugs. In a clinical setting, supplying a drug for patient use is commonly referred to as 'dispensing'.

If 'Patient G' needs to have a specific drug to treat their condition, this drug first needs to be prescribed for them, then it has to be supplied to the clinical area and finally it has to be administered to Patient G by someone.

Prescribing a drug for Patient G's use means that the prescriber authorises, in writing, another person to supply a specific drug at a specific dose for a set period of time for use by Patient G.

Supplying or dispensing a drug occurs when an authorised individual provides the actual drug in the correct dose and quantity for the patient's use. Depending on the circumstances, the drug may be supplied directly to the patient or to a clinical area for administration to the patient. The dispensing of a drug goes beyond supply as it involves ensuring that the prescription is valid and that the drug is appropriate for the individual patient and will not adversely interact with other drugs that the patient may be taking.

Administering a drug involves the physical act of providing the drug to the patient or supervising the patient taking the drug. This includes checking that the correct patient is going to receive the correct dose of the correct drug at the correct time and via the correct route. The route includes oral, injection, through skin contact or via insertion into an orifice.

All three activities that precede a patient taking a drug are regulated in some form or other. Only certain groups of individuals may undertake each of the activities. Until the early 1990s, for a patient in a hospital, this would have been the doctor who prescribed the drug, the pharmacist who supplied/dispensed it and the nurse who administered it.

Do drugs have to be destroyed in certain ways?

There are times when individual patients may no longer require a prescribed drug, maybe because they have been prescribed another drug, or have left the clinical area or have recovered from the condition that the drug was prescribed for. Unless the patient was being administered drugs from a general supply, as opposed to having a supply in their own name, this may mean that there is a quantity of drugs within the clinical area that no longer need to be administered to that patient. Something has to be done with these drugs, but what?

Where there is a supply of drugs for a named patient, the drug should not be used for other patients without the authorisation of the person who supplied/ dispensed the drug. There may be specific aspects of the drug's formulation, which can mean it is appropriate for one patient but inappropriate for another.

Your employer should have a policy for dealing with drugs that are no longer required. You should consult this where possible. Best practice would be to either return the drug to the supplier, or to have them collect the excess drugs from your clinical area, as they will know whether they can be reused, or if not, they will arrange for the safe destruction of the drugs.

If the drug is a controlled drug, it may only be destroyed by someone who is an 'authorised person' (The Misuse of Drugs Regulations 2001: Section 27), or on their directions. There are specific mechanisms for the destruction of controlled drugs and for the recording of their destruction.

Where drugs are removed from the stock of a clinical area, this needs to be recorded, along with where they were returned to or how they were destroyed.

Can patients self-administer their drugs in a clinical setting?

Until it was withdrawn on 28th January 2019, the Nursing and Midwifery Council (NMC) had guidance in its *Standards for Medicines Management* (Nursing and Midwifery Council, 2017) in relation to self-administration of drugs by patients. The guidance has been withdrawn because the NMC no longer believes that they should be providing clinical guidance in this area and not because they do not see this as a useful feature of clinical practice.

Provided that the patient is competent to do so, in most cases there is no reason why patients cannot be allowed to self-administer their drugs when they are in a clinical setting. Indeed, having patients self-administer their drugs increases the role they can play in their own healthcare and may provide a degree of control that could otherwise be lacking.

There is a spectrum of self-administration that patients may undertake ranging from the healthcare practitioner being in charge of the drugs but allowing the patient to access them when required and supervising the administration, through the healthcare practitioner just supervising the administration of the drug, to the patient taking sole responsibility for all aspects of the drug, including its storage and administration.

Patients should only self-administer their drugs when they want to do so. Whilst this can be encouraged, it should not be enforced on a patient as this may affect their compliance with their drug regimen.

Your employer should have guidance on whether or when patients can be allowed to self-administer their drugs. Where self-administration by patients is allowed, the guidance should provide detail as to how this can be undertaken and any specific documentation that would need to be completed. In the absence of any guidance, before allowing a patient to self-administer their drugs, the healthcare practitioner should check that the patient knows:

- the drugs they need to self-administer
- the times that each drug needs to be taken
- the dose of each drug to be taken and how many tablets this is, or where it is a cream, for example, how much of the cream to use on each occasion
- how long they need to continue taking the drug
- whether and, if so how, they need to record the taking of the drug
- about any side effects, what to look out for and what to do if a side effect may have occurred
- where to seek assistance, guidance and information if it is needed.

Many healthcare practitioners may be wary of allowing patients to self-administer their drugs because they believe that they are liable for the patient's actions and they will face consequences if a patient forgets to self-administer their drugs or makes an error in taking a drug. However, provided that the healthcare practitioner has followed any local guidance on patient self-administration of drugs, ensures that the patient is competent to self-administer their drugs and has the necessary information to do so, this would not be the case, as the patient would be liable for their own actions where they voluntarily self-administer their drugs.

Is it ever appropriate to give a patient their drugs covertly?

If a patient is competent (see **How is competence assessed?** [p. 71]), then they have the right to decide what treatment to consent to and what to refuse; this includes taking drugs. If a competent patient refuses to take drugs, that should be respected. It is acceptable to explain why the drug has been prescribed for them and any consequences of not taking it. If the competent patient continues to refuse to take the drug, this is their decision and it is not legally or ethically acceptable to covertly give them the drug.

The only time when it is acceptable and appropriate to give patients their drugs covertly is when they lack the competence to make decisions regarding their drug treatment. This could be because they are a child or because they have been assessed as lacking competence using the criteria in the Mental Capacity Act 2005.

Before turning to covertly administering drugs, it may be appropriate to approach family members to see if they can assist in persuading patients to take their drugs normally, although patient confidentiality will need to be maintained.

Where a patient, who lacks competence to make their own decisions regarding their drug therapy, refuses to take drugs that are considered to be an essential part of their treatment and to take the drug(s) would be in their best interests, and the patient cannot be persuaded to take the drug, and no other method of providing the drug such as in an alternative formulation, for example liquid instead of a pill, is available, then, and only then, can the drug be given to the patient covertly.

Of course, if the patient has an advance decision in place (see **What is a living will or advance decision? [p. 88]**) that specifically excludes the covert administration of drugs, this needs to be followed.

Before drugs are administered to a patient covertly, the healthcare practitioner needs to consider whether it is necessary to consult with the patient's relatives, and this would be best practice where a relative or other individual has lasting power of attorney for a patient's decision making in relation to their health.

Administration of drugs by covert means should be the exception rather than the norm and never undertaken for the convenience of healthcare practitioners. Any clinical area that endorses the covert administration of drugs to patients should have a transparent policy in place that explains when this may happen and how it will be undertaken.

Documenting any instance of the covert administration of drugs in the relevant patient's health record is essential. If it will be an ongoing situation, this also needs to be recorded, along with the decision-making process that led to this decision.

The most common way of giving a drug covertly is to do so by disguising it in the patient's food or drink. Before disguising the drug in the food or drink, advice needs to be obtained from a suitable healthcare practitioner, such as a pharmacist, as to whether the specific food or drink may have an unintended effect on the drug.

Can I use drugs from the ward drugs cupboard for my personal use?

Taking something without the consent of the owner can be considered theft, which is a criminal offence and could result in the healthcare practitioner facing a criminal charge, an employer disciplinary hearing and a fitness to practise investigation by their regulatory body.

Unless you wish to possibly face these consequences, do not take any drugs from a clinical area unless you have permission to do so.

Your employer may have a policy that permits staff using clinical supplies for their personal needs. If they don't, do not take anything for your personal use, the possible consequences are not worth it. If there is a policy, do consult this before taking anything; the policy should say what can be taken for personal use, for example paracetamol but not antibiotics, and also who can authorise drugs being taken for personal use. If there is a specific individual who needs to give permission, contact that person for authorisation before taking anything for your own use and ensure that this is documented appropriately.

Q **What should I do if asked by a senior healthcare practitioner to administer a drug that is not included in my employer's protocols?**

A For a discussion of delegation, see **How does delegation affect liability? (p. 53).**

If a drug is not included in your employer's protocol, this suggests that your employer does not want you to administer it.

It may be that you and other healthcare practitioners at your role or level are prohibited from administering the particular drug, but other levels of healthcare practitioner can, or it may be a blanket prohibition. If it is the former, you should inform the senior healthcare practitioner of this fact and politely decline as you are not authorised, and suggest that they or other healthcare practitioners could administer the drug under the protocol. If it is the latter, you should inform the senior healthcare practitioner that your employer does not permit the administration of this particular drug and they should contact someone for further guidance.

You should not administer the drug yourself and should use your employer's protocol to support your position. If necessary, you could contact your manager or other senior person to intervene on your behalf with the senior healthcare practitioner.

Q **If possession of a controlled drug is unlawful, am I able to transport them to a patient in the community?**

A There is a fallacy amongst some healthcare practitioners that, because the possession of controlled drugs is restricted, the provisions in the Misuse of Drugs Act 1971 mean that a healthcare practitioner is not allowed to possess them or transport them to a patient for administration; and that if they did, they could face a criminal prosecution.

Whilst this is true for members of the public, The Misuse of Drugs Regulations 2001 makes provision for certain types of individual to prescribe, supply and possess controlled drugs according to which Schedule they belong to. Thus, The Misuse of Drugs Regulations 2001, specifically Section 6(7), gives the healthcare practitioner a defence against prosecution, provided they follow the legal requirements for each type of controlled drug.

So, if a healthcare practitioner can prescribe a controlled drug, the provisions in The Misuse of Drugs Regulations 2001 mean that they are also allowed to transport it to a patient.

Additionally, Section 7 of The Misuse of Drugs Regulations 2001 gives a blanket authority to any healthcare practitioner acting under the authority of a doctor or dentist to administer a controlled drug in Schedules 2, 3 or 4, even if they would not otherwise have authority in their own right. The right to administer also includes the right to possess the controlled drug for the purpose of that administration and this includes the right to transport it to the place of administration.

Although healthcare practitioners are legally entitled to possess and transport controlled drugs in certain circumstances, this does not mean that they can just carry them as a matter of routine in case a patient needs them. The controlled drug in question needs to be for a specific named patient.

This does not apply to doctors and dentists who have authority under The Misuse of Drugs Regulations 2001 to possess and supply controlled drugs, and may provide these to patients, for instance a general practitioner on a home visit. There is also an exemption for midwives in Section 11 of The Misuse of Drugs Regulations 2001 with regard to the possession of certain controlled drugs, whereby they can possess controlled drugs without them being for a named patient under certain circumstances. The Controlled Drugs (Supervision of Management and Use) Regulations 2013 authorises paramedics to possess and administer controlled drugs for non-named patients.

Section 6(2) of The Misuse of Drugs Regulations 2001 allows healthcare practitioners to remove controlled drugs from a patient's home when they are no longer required and to transport them to a place for their destruction, for example a hospital, general practitioner surgery or a pharmacy.

Any healthcare practitioner who needs to possess controlled drugs outside of a permanent clinical area would be well advised to ensure that they know their employer's policy on the possession and transport of controlled drugs, including any requirements on recording their actions. Although the law may allow you to possess and transport controlled drugs, your employer may not, so it is always good to check before proceeding.

What limits a healthcare practitioner's ability to prescribe drugs?

Traditionally, it was only doctors and dentists who had a legal right to prescribe prescription only medicines. This was recognised in the Medicines Act 1968 where Section 58 specifically states that only doctors and dentists are appropriate practitioners in relation to the provisions in the Act. Interestingly, the section also includes veterinary surgeons and veterinary practitioners as appropriate practitioners but that is in relation to animals and so outside the scope of our discussion.

So rather than indicating who is not permitted to prescribe, the Act defines the class of individuals, known as 'appropriate practitioners', who are permitted to prescribe prescription only medicines.

In more recent years, the definition of 'appropriate practitioners' has widened to include members of other healthcare practitioner groups.

Anyone who breaches Section 58 of the Medicines Act 1968, by prescribing drugs when they are not authorised to do so, could face a criminal prosecution.

Q Which healthcare practitioner groups can prescribe?

A Doctors and dentists are the traditional prescribers, although dentists are only allowed to prescribe from a limited dental practitioners' formulary. Any other group of healthcare practitioners who are now able to prescribe come under the overall heading of 'non-medical prescribing'.

Various healthcare practitioner groups have gained the right to prescribe at different times. The following is the current alphabetical list of those healthcare practitioner groups who have the right to prescribe:

- chiropodists
- dentists
- dietitians
- doctors
- midwives
- nurses
- optometrists
- paramedics
- pharmacists
- physiotherapists
- podiatrists
- radiographers.

It should be noted that not every healthcare practitioner in all the groups has the right to prescribe. Members of some of the healthcare practitioner groups have to undergo specific training in order to obtain the right to prescribe. There are also different categories of prescriber and different lists of medicinal products (formularies) that they are allowed to prescribe from.

Q What types of prescriber are there?

A Legislation currently provides for three types of prescriber. These are:

- community practitioner nurse prescribers
- independent prescribers, and
- supplementary prescribers.

All forms of prescribing are an extension to the normal role of the healthcare practitioner on initial registration.

COMMUNITY PRACTITIONER NURSE PRESCRIBERS

This was the first group of non-medical prescribers. Their authorisation comes from the Medicinal Products: Prescription by Nurses etc. Act 1992.

These prescribers are nurses who have been registered with the Nursing and Midwifery Council for at least two years before successfully completing a Community Practitioner Nurse Prescribing course (also known as V100 or V150 courses).

As may be guessed from their title, Community Practitioner Nurse prescribers are nurses who work within the community rather than in a hospital or other such setting. They include district nurses, community nurses, health visitors and school nurses.

Community Practitioner Nurse prescribers are only able to prescribe from a limited formulary known as the 'Nurse Prescribers' Formulary for Community Practitioners', usually shortened to the 'Nurse Prescribers' Formulary' (or NPF) and previously known as 'The Nurse Prescribers' Formulary for District Nurses and Health Visitors'. The Nurse Prescribers' Formulary is based on what may be needed in a community setting such as dressings, appliances and drugs from the General Sale List (GSL) and Pharmacy list (P) and a very limited number of drugs from the Prescription Only Medicines (POM) list.

INDEPENDENT PRESCRIBERS

The Health and Social Care Act 2001, specifically Section 63, contained provision for the extension of non-medical prescribing to groups other than community-based nurses and an extension of what could be prescribed. A new formulary was introduced, the Nurse Prescribers' Extended Formulary, hence their original name of Extended Formulary Nurse Prescribers. This allowed the prescriber to prescribe any drug on the GSL or P lists and the number of POMs was increased; but prescribing was limited to four types of conditions:

- minor ailments
- minor injuries
- health promotion
- palliative care.

In 2006, the restriction on prescribing for the four conditions was removed and, with the exception of some controlled and unlicensed drugs, the prescriber was able to prescribe from the whole of the British National Formulary.

The current situation, which started in April 2012, is that an independent prescriber, who is registered with the relevant regulatory body as an independent prescriber (which would include a note on the register to this effect) is able to prescribe any drug from the British National Formulary that is within their sphere of competence, including controlled drugs.

Independent prescribers, which is a term that now includes both the traditional prescribers, doctors and dentists, and the new independent prescribers described above, have liability for assessing the patient's clinical need, making a diagnosis and formulating a treatment plan, which may include prescribing.

SUPPLEMENTARY PRESCRIBERS

Although the Health and Social Care Act 2001 introduced supplementary prescribing, it required other legislation before it became a reality. In 2003, The National Health Service (Amendments Relating to Prescribing by Nurses and Pharmacists etc.) (England) Regulations 2003 provided that legislative authority. It was later in the same year that the first courses were available for supplementary prescribers.

Initially, supplementary prescribers were known as 'dependent prescribers' and this may be a more accurate term for the way they are allowed to prescribe. Whilst an independent prescriber can assess and diagnose a patient, and make a treatment plan, including the prescription of drugs, a supplementary prescriber cannot.

Supplementary prescribers provide ongoing care to patients after they have been assessed and received a diagnosis and treatment plan from an independent prescriber. Once a clinical treatment/management plan has been agreed between the independent and supplementary prescriber, the supplementary prescriber may prescribe any drug that is noted in the clinical treatment plan from the whole of the British National Formulary, including controlled drugs, that are clinically necessary.

Supplementary prescribers are dependent upon the independent prescriber to undertake the initial stages of the patient's treatment needs, hence the original term of dependent prescriber. A supplementary prescriber takes over the care and treatment of the patient once a clinical treatment plan has been agreed and is often involved in the treatment of long-term conditions where there is a need for continued assessment, repeat prescriptions and possible alteration of drug dose.

Supplementary prescribing is related to specific named patients and the clinical treatment plan must be for that specific patient.

As an independent prescriber, is it OK for me to prescribe drugs for my family members?

There is no law in the United Kingdom that prohibits an independent prescriber from prescribing for themselves or for a family member. However, it is an ethical minefield and generally considered to be unethical practice to do so by most of the regulatory bodies. For instance, in its 'Good medical practice' document, the General Medical Council states, 'wherever possible, avoid providing medical care to yourself or anyone with whom you have a close personal relationship' (General Medical Council, 2013: paragraph 16g). In this context, medical care explicitly includes prescribing.

Objectivity is a major reason why it is not considered a safe practice to prescribe for oneself or family members. Most healthcare practitioners are likely to find it difficult to be objective about their own health needs, let alone their family members. Without objectivity in prescribing, unsafe or unsuitable prescribing can occur.

This is also an issue of confidentiality. If a healthcare practitioner were to prescribe for themselves, at least they already know their confidential health information and they can maintain the confidentiality of that information. It is questionable whether a family member would want to share all their past medical history with a relative, even if they were a healthcare practitioner. Without access to their relative's health record, the prescriber cannot check for information that the patient doesn't recall, which would be relevant to the intended prescription. If the prescriber does not have access to all the relevant information, this can lead to inappropriate prescribing and possibly drug interactions.

If a healthcare practitioner were to prescribe for a family member, they would be interposing themselves between the relative and the relative's usual healthcare practitioner. This raises the issue of how the relative's usual healthcare practitioner would gain access to the information about the prescribing so that they are aware of it for any future healthcare needs and continuity of care. Additionally, record keeping of the prescribing incident would need to be considered.

When prescribing for a family member, consideration needs to be given to what happens if something untoward were to occur, for instance a drug reaction. How would this be managed and who might the family member have redress against?

Prescribing for a family member puts you in an invidious position. The only circumstances in which it can be ethically justified is when it is life-saving treatment or where delay would be detrimental to the family member. This would be where for some reason the family member cannot attend their usual prescriber and receive a prescription from them, and there is no alternative other than for you to prescribe the necessary drugs.

As a non-prescriber, what can I do in relation to the prescribing of drugs to patients?

The previous questions in this chapter have demonstrated that the prescribing of drugs is legally regulated and can only be undertaken by certain groups of individuals.

Likewise, the supply of drugs to patients is also regulated and must be carried out by authorised individuals.

The main role of a healthcare practitioner who is a non-prescriber is in the administration of drugs to a patient. Although it needs to be remembered that even the administration of drugs is something that is regulated, especially for controlled drugs and certain other categories of drugs. Therefore, even though a healthcare practitioner does not need to be a prescriber to administer drugs to a patient, any healthcare practitioner involved in the administration of drugs to patients needs to ensure that they have the appropriate training for the particular drug and route of administration.

Q

What is a Patient Group Direction and is it a form of prescribing?

A

Patient Group Directions (PGDs) have existed for longer than independent prescribers, although they have been known by different names throughout the years. The Prescription Only Medicines (Human Use) Amendment Order 2000 made amendments to the then existing legislation to allow PGDs to be used.

A PGD is a protocol that allows certain named drugs to be supplied and/or administered to a patient, who does not need to be named or identified, in a specified group with an identified clinical condition and/or in a specific clinical situation without the need for an individual prescription to be written and signed by a doctor or dentist. The drugs that can be administered using a PGD include prescription only medicines and some controlled drugs.

The idea behind PGD is that they make use of healthcare practitioners' skills to maximise the use of resources and reduce the time that patients access treatment.

As may be expected, there are rules relating to the writing and use of PGDs. They need to be written by a doctor and pharmacist and in collaboration with the healthcare practitioners who will be using them. They also need to be authorised by a senior doctor and senior pharmacist, and ratified by the relevant health organisation, for example the National Health Service (NHS) Trust. It is recommended that all healthcare practitioners who are approved to use the PGD are named in it and also sign it to indicate that they agree with it. PGDs should be reviewed at least every two years.

The Prescription Only Medicines (Human Use) Amendment Order 2000 detailed the particulars that have to be included in a PGD. These are:

a) the period during which the Direction shall have effect;
b) the description or class of prescription only medicine to which the Direction relates;
c) whether there are any restrictions on the quantity of medicine which may be supplied on any one occasion, and, if so, what restrictions;

d)   the clinical situations which prescription only medicines of that description or class may be used to treat;

e)   the clinical criteria under which a person shall be eligible for treatment;

f)   whether any class of person is excluded from treatment under the Direction and, if so, what class of person;

g)   whether there are circumstances in which further advice should be sought from a doctor or dentist and, if so, what circumstances;

h)   the pharmaceutical form or forms in which prescription only medicines of that description or class are to be administered;

i)   the strength, or maximum strength, at which prescription only medicines of that description or class are to be administered;

j)   the applicable dosage or maximum dosage;

k)   the route of administration;

l)   the frequency of administration;

m) any minimum or maximum period of administration applicable to prescription only medicines of that description or class;

n)   whether there are any relevant warnings to note, and, if so, what warnings;

o)   whether there is any follow up action to be taken in any circumstances, and, if so, what action and in what circumstances;

p)   arrangements for referral for medical advice;

q)   details of the records to be kept of the supply, or the administration, of medicines under the Direction (The Prescription Only Medicines [Human Use] Amendment Order 2000: Schedule 7).

Currently, it is the Human Medicines Regulations 2012 that governs the use of PGDs (the above particulars from the 2000 Order are included in this Regulation).

It is important to note that only the named healthcare practitioners can administer the named drugs within the PGD to patients. If the PGD allows, healthcare practitioners can adjust the dose of a drug according to the clinical need of a specific patient.

PGDs mean that patients with specific clinical needs and/or conditions can be seen by healthcare practitioners and receive the treatment they need within the clinical guidelines as set out in the PGDs, without the need for a prescription or an assessment by a prescriber. They are not meant to be used as a substitute for individualised patient care, and should only be used where their use would be advantageous for patients and would not compromise patient safety.

There is no requirement that a healthcare practitioner approved to use a PGD undertakes any prescribing training. This is because the healthcare practitioners who use a PGD are not considered to be prescribing as they are acting under the direction of the doctor and pharmacist who wrote the PGD. Indeed, this is an additional role that the non-prescriber can undertake.

Q Is there an agreed prescribing standard?

A The standard that a prescriber has to meet in their prescribing practice is the same as that discussed when considering **What is the legal standard I have to reach in my practice? (p. 46)**. This is the standard required by the 'Bolam test', as modified by the 'Bolitho test', of the ordinary competent prescriber.

This means that a prescriber needs to ensure they have the necessary knowledge and skills, and that their prescribing practice is evidence based, capable of withstanding logical scrutiny and in line with practice as demonstrated by ordinary competent prescribers within their specific speciality and profession.

That said, the regulatory bodies provide some guidance on prescribing and the standard expected. The Health and Care Professions Council and the Nursing and Midwifery Council have adopted the Royal Pharmaceutical Society's guidance on prescribing standards, *A Competency Framework for all Prescribers* (2016); whilst the General Medical Council continues to issue their own guidance, *Good practice on prescribing and managing devices* (2013).

To meet the 'Bolam test', a healthcare practitioner would need to demonstrate that their prescribing practice was safe and adhered to the guidance from the relevant regulatory body. There is also a need to consider whether the prescriber's employer has any guidance or policies in place relating to prescribing practice, and if so, the prescriber would need to follow this as well. Any departure from accepted guidance and practice would need to have a very strong reason that is logical and defensible.

As well as meeting the required standard at any one point in time, the prescribing healthcare practitioner needs to be able to demonstrate how they keep their prescribing practice up to date and how they maintain their competence to prescribe.

SUMMARY

- A drug is a substance that has an effect on the body.
- Drugs are categorised into three classes so that their sale and supply can be restricted where necessary.
- Controlled drugs are those drugs whose activities, such as supply and possession, are controlled and subject to restrictions; breaching these is a criminal offence.
- Before a patient receives a drug in a clinical setting, it has to be prescribed, supplied and administered to them.
- Removal of drugs from the stock of a clinical area needs to be recorded. Controlled drugs can only be destroyed by authorised persons or on their directions.
- Provided that the patient is competent to do so, they may self-administer their drugs in a clinical area.
- Drugs may be given to patients covertly in very specific circumstances, but not to competent patients.

- Do not take any drugs from a clinical area for your own use unless you have express permission to do so from someone authorised to give permission.
- You should not administer drugs that are not included in your employer's protocols, even if asked to do so by a senior healthcare practitioner.
- Healthcare practitioners are legally allowed to possess and transport controlled drugs in certain circumstances.
- Traditionally, only doctors and dentists were appropriate practitioners allowed to prescribe prescription only medicines. The definition of 'appropriate practitioners' has widened in recent years.
- There are currently three types of prescriber:
  - community practitioner nurse prescribers
  - independent prescribers, and
  - supplementary prescribers.
- Unless it is an emergency, it is not considered good practice to prescribe for oneself or for family members, or others with whom the prescriber has a close personal relationship.
- The role of non-prescribers in relation to the prescribing of drugs to patients is in their administration.
- Patient Group Directions (PGDs) allow named healthcare practitioners to supply and administer named drugs in specified situations to patients with an identified clinical need/condition. PGDs are not a form of prescribing and non-prescribers can be authorised to use them.
- Prescribers need to meet the standard of the ordinary competent prescriber in their prescribing practice.

REFERENCES

General Medical Council (2013) *Good Medical Practice*. General Medical Council: London.
General Medical Council (2013) *Good practice on prescribing and managing devices*. General Medical Council: London.
Health and Social Care Act 2001.
Human Medicines Regulations 2012 (SI 2012/1916).
Medicinal Products: Prescription by Nurses etc. Act 1992.
Medicines Act 1968.
Mental Capacity Act 2005.
Misuse of Drugs Act 1971.
Nursing and Midwifery Council (2017) *Standards for Medicines Management*. Nursing and Midwifery Council: London.
Royal Pharmaceutical Society (2016) *A Competency Framework for all Prescribers*. Royal Pharmaceutical Society: London.
The Controlled Drugs (Supervision of Management and Use) Regulations 2013 (SI 2013/373).
The Misuse of Drugs Regulations 2001 (SI 2001/3998).
The National Health Service (Amendments Relating to Prescribing by Nurses and Pharmacists etc.) (England) Regulations 2003 (SI 2003/699).
The Prescription Only Medicines (Human Use) Amendment Order 2000 (SI 2000/1917).

REPRODUCTION AND PARENTING

This chapter is concerned with the legal and ethical aspects of reproduction, and who may act in the parental role and make decisions for the care and treatment of a child.

Reproductive issues from a legal and ethical perspective are those concerned with pre-conception and conception, through to the removal of the foetus from the body, whether naturally or due to medical intervention. This chapter develops this further and encompasses questions relating to the parentage of the resultant child.

QUESTIONS COVERED IN CHAPTER 8

- Why do healthcare practitioners need to know about reproductive and parenting issues?
- Is abortion legal?
- What is the legal status of the foetus?
- Whose legal rights are paramount, the foetus' or the mother's?
- Whose legal rights are paramount, the prospective mother's or father's?
- What is surrogacy?
- When can a healthcare practitioner conscientiously object to take part in a patient's treatment?
- Who is a parent and who has parental responsibility?
- Are children allowed to make decisions regarding their reproductive health?

 Why do healthcare practitioners need to know about reproductive and parenting issues?

 Reproductive issues are not confined to a single area of healthcare. Rather, the legal and ethical issues in reproductive healthcare practice resonate across many areas of healthcare and many healthcare practitioners may come across these issues even when they work outside of what may be seen as reproductive healthcare practice. These may be patients who are acting as surrogates for another person or who need to receive care and treatment following a termination of pregnancy. Having knowledge of the legal and ethical issues can be beneficial in providing care and treatment for these patients.

In a similar way, many healthcare practitioners who do not work within traditional child-focused areas of healthcare may need to interact with children during their practice. Some of these children will have parents who are not their natural parents, for example because they were born as a result of a surrogacy arrangement, have been adopted or are in care. Being aware of the legal distinction between a natural parent and who has parental responsibility (see **Who is a parent and who has parental responsibility? [p. 180]**) for a child is essential when caring and treating a child. It allows the healthcare practitioner to know who to approach for any decisions that need to be made on the child's behalf.

Q

Is abortion legal?

A

This is a controversial area in reproductive health, it is fraught with religious, moral and ethical issues and debates. These will not be discussed here other than acknowledging that some healthcare practitioners may have a conscientious objection to taking part in abortions (see **When can a healthcare practitioner conscientiously object to take part in a patient's treatment? [p. 179]**).

Abortion has been a criminal offence since the 1200s when it was a common law offence that was triable in the ecclesiastical courts. It was not until 1803 that it first appeared as an offence in a statute, the Malicious Shooting or Stabbing Act 1803. Although this Act was concerned with individuals causing, or intending to cause, a pregnant woman to have an abortion.

With the introduction of the Offences Against the Person Act 1861, Section 58, the pregnant woman could also be charged with a criminal offence for procuring or attempting to procure an abortion. Section 58 makes it a criminal offence for a woman to take a substance to procure an abortion (called a 'miscarriage' in the Act) or to use an instrument or other means to do the same. It also makes it a criminal offence for someone else to procure a woman's abortion. Section 59 of the Act makes it a criminal offence to obtain and/or supply the means for causing an abortion.

Following the introduction of the Offences Against the Person Act 1861, one thing that was unclear was whether it was permissible to cause an abortion in order to preserve the life of the pregnant woman. A 1939 court case concluded that there was a common law defence to the criminal offence of abortion (R v Bourne, where a doctor performed an abortion on a 14-year-old girl who had been raped by five soldiers and was acquitted of the offence on the basis of saving the life of the girl).

For a crime to be committed, three things must exist; there has to be a criminal act, a criminal intent and an absence of a legal defence. So, although someone may undertake an abortion and intend its consequences, if they have a lawful reason for doing so (i.e. they have a legal defence), they will not be committing a criminal offence.

Sections 58 and 59 of the Offences Against the Person Act 1861 remain in force today and form the basis of the law criminalising abortion. At the time of writing, abortion remains a criminal offence.

This statement requires us to consider the provisions of the Abortion Act 1967, for many people, including many healthcare practitioners, believe that the Act legalises abortion, which it doesn't. Neither does it provide a woman with the right to demand an abortion. What the Abortion Act 1967 actually does is to provide a defence to the criminal law on abortion. It may be worth noting the full title of the Act, which is 'An Act to amend and clarify the law relating to termination of pregnancy by registered medical practitioners'. This is exactly what it does.

The Abortion Act 1967 provides the circumstances under which an abortion may be lawfully performed. These are very specific and, if they are not followed exactly, an abortion would still be a criminal offence.

For an abortion to be considered lawful, Section 1(1) of the Abortion Act 1967 requires that two registered medical practitioners (doctors) must be of the opinion:

a) that the pregnancy has not exceeded its twenty-fourth week and that the continuance of the pregnancy would involve risk, greater than if the pregnancy were terminated, of injury to the physical or mental health of the pregnant woman or any existing children of her family; or

b) that the termination is necessary to prevent grave permanent injury to the physical or mental health of the pregnant woman; or

c) that the continuance of the pregnancy would involve risk to the life of the pregnant woman, greater than if the pregnancy were terminated; or

d) that there is a substantial risk that if the child were born it would suffer from such physical or mental abnormalities as to be seriously handicapped.

There is also a requirement (Section 1[3]) that the termination of pregnancy is carried out in a designated place such as an approved hospital or clinic.

Section 1(4) of the Abortion Act 1967 allows for 'the termination of a pregnancy by a registered medical practitioner in a case where he is of the opinion, formed in good faith, that the termination is immediately necessary to save the life or to prevent grave permanent injury to the physical or mental health of the pregnant woman'. The difference to Section 1(1) is that where a termination of pregnancy is immediately necessary, only one doctor needs to assess the patient.

Section 2 of the Abortion Act 1967 requires notice of terminations of pregnancy to be provided to the relevant authorities.

Save for the exemption and defence to a criminal offence in the specific circumstances set out in the Abortion Act 1967, abortion remains a criminal offence. This means that a woman has no automatic right to an abortion because two registered medical practitioners have to form an opinion that the abortion is justified on one of the grounds listed in the Abortion Act 1967, Section 1.

Q What is the legal status of the foetus?

A For the purposes of this chapter, a 'foetus' is defined as being the product of human conception from its eighth week of existence to the time of its birth. Prior to the eighth week, it is termed an 'embryo'.

To have legal status within English law, the thing in question needs to have a legal personality. The existence of legal personality permits someone or something to exercise legal rights. This means that someone with a legal personality can claim legal rights and can take legal action to protect those rights.

The embryo has some legal protection by virtue of its recognition within the provisions of the Human Fertilisation and Embryology Act 1990; although this protection does not go as far as establishing that the embryo has a legal personality.

Section 3 of the Human Fertilisation and Embryology Act 1990 prohibits certain activities, such as placing a human embryo in an animal, and licences certain other activities such as their storage. Once an embryo has attained its primitive streak, all activities are prohibited. Section 3(4) states, 'the primitive streak is to be taken to have appeared in an embryo not later than the end of the period of 14 days beginning with the day on which the process of creating the embryo began'. This means that once an embryo has reached 14 days, it cannot be subject to further research.

The foetus is not recognised as having legal personality until it has an existence that is independent of its mother. In the case of Re MB [1997] (see **How can a healthcare practitioner lawfully treat an incompetent patient? [p. 91]** for the Case Note), it was stated, 'a foetus, up to the moment of birth, does not have any separate interest capable of being taken into account by a court' (Re MB [[1997]: 176).

There may be said to be an oddity on the law in that, although the foetus has no legal personality until it has an independent existence, once it attains an independent existence, its legal personality is almost backdated to cover the period when it was dependent upon its mother.

The Attorney-General's Reference No. 3 of 1994 (a case which had to decide if a man who stabbed his girlfriend and unborn child, which died after being born prematurely, should be charged with murder or manslaughter) confirmed that, if a foetus had an independent existence of its mother but subsequently dies as a result of injuries caused to it whilst it was dependent upon the mother in her womb, for instance if the mother was assaulted, the mother's assailant could be charged with manslaughter of the baby rather than just assault of the mother.

Similarly, the child can sue for injuries caused to it whilst it was dependent upon the mother in her womb, where the injury was a result of a breach of duty owed to the mother (Congenital Disabilities [Civil Liability] Act 1976).

Thus, although the foetus is not legally recognised as having a separate legal existence and legal personality until it has an existence independent of its mother, once it has attained its legal personality, its rights in both civil and criminal law are retrospectively applied (Cornock and Montgomery, 2011).

Q

Whose legal rights are paramount, the foetus' or the mother's?

A

It was noted earlier in this chapter (when considering **What is the legal status of the foetus? [p. 176]**) that the foetus has no legal personality until it has an independent existence of its mother. Until that time, the law recognises that a competent woman is entitled to make decisions for her own body including those that affect the foetus. From an ethical perspective the woman would be said to have complete self-determination over her body, even if the decisions she makes are detrimental to the foetus.

Legally, if the health needs of the woman and the foetus are in conflict, the consent of a competent woman is sufficient for any decision relating to her body even where this adversely affects the foetus.

A healthcare practitioner cannot make a treatment decision based upon the needs of the foetus where a competent woman disagrees with the planned course of action.

It has been established in common law that 'a competent woman may choose, even for irrational reasons, not to have medical intervention, even though the consequences may be the death of, or serious handicap to, the child she bears; or her own life' (Re MB [1997]: 175) (see **How can a healthcare practitioner lawfully treat an incompetent patient? [p. 91]** for the Case Note).

If the woman is incompetent to make decisions, any treatment decisions need to be made in their best interests, not those of the foetus.

Equally, if a child were born who had suffered demonstrable harm as a result of something that the mother did during her pregnancy, for instance smoking, drinking excessively or taking illegal drugs, the child would not be able to bring an action against the mother for the harm suffered. This is because the mother does not have any legal liability to the foetus until it has an independent existence. The liability of the mother, which cannot be backdated, contrasts with the civil and criminal liability owed to the foetus by others, which can be backdated once the foetus attains its own legal personality.

Q

Whose legal rights are paramount, the prospective mother's or father's?

A

In relation to the unborn child, previous questions in this chapter have already noted that the foetus is considered to be a part of the woman's body and, if that woman is competent, she may make a decision regarding her body even if they could be detrimental to the foetus.

Based upon this, it should come as no surprise that from a legal perspective the woman's decision is paramount and the prospective father has no legal right to make any decisions over the woman's body for the benefit of the foetus. Indeed, they do not even have a right to be consulted over decisions without the mother's consent.

Q What is surrogacy?

A Surrogacy is when one woman enters into agreement to carry a baby for another person or couple with the intention of giving that baby to them at birth. Whilst surrogacy is legal in the United Kingdom, there are various aspects that need to be carefully navigated in order that the particular surrogacy does not become unlawful.

The Surrogacy Arrangements Act 1985 prohibits anyone advertising that they are willing to be a surrogate or that they are looking for a surrogate mother; although the Act makes an exemption for non-profit organisations. It is also an offence for a third party to be involved in a surrogacy arrangement or for payment to be made to a surrogate mother other than for their expenses (such as loss of earnings, medical expenses and expenses related to the pregnancy).

In order for the surrogacy to be legal, there needs to be a surrogacy arrangement put in place before the surrogate mother becomes pregnant. However, under Section 1A of the Surrogacy Arrangements Act 1985, a surrogacy arrangement is not enforceable in law and either side may withdraw from the arrangement.

There are two forms of surrogacy, one where the intended parents supply the egg and have it fertilised before it is placed into the surrogate mother so that she has no genetic link to the baby, and the second where eggs from the surrogate mother are used, and fertilised by the intended father, so that she does have a genetic link to the baby.

One issue that can be legally difficult is who the legal parents of a child born through surrogacy are. The law in the United Kingdom recognises that the surrogate mother who carries and gives birth to the baby is the legal mother of the baby even if they have no genetic link to it. Parentage will be considered further in **Who is a parent and who has parental responsibility?** (p. 180).

If the intended parents want to be the baby's legally recognised parents, they need to apply to either adopt the child or for a parental order, which can be granted by the Courts. This is the case even if the surrogacy occurred outside of the United Kingdom and the baby is brought back to reside in the United Kingdom. The Human Fertilisation and Embryology Act 2008 has strict criteria that must be followed for a parental order to be granted, such as:

- one of the parents applying for the parental order has to be the biological parent, i.e. have a genetic link to the baby
- the child must be living with the applicants
- the parental order must be applied for within six months of the child's birth

- the applicants must be at least 18
- the surrogate mother consents to the making of the order
- the court must be satisfied that only expenses have been paid to the surrogate mother, and
- since 3rd January 2019, one parent has been allowed to apply for a parental order; before that it had to be a couple, although they did not have to be married or in a civil partnership.

When can a healthcare practitioner conscientiously object to take part in a patient's treatment?

'Conscientious objection' 'is a phrase which can be utilised in two ways. The first use relates to an individual who raises a moral reason for not undertaking a specific action. The second mode of use is that where there is a legal conscience clause which creates an opt-out category for individuals from a specific duty' (Cornock, 2008: 7).

In healthcare, conscientious objection is the mechanism whereby healthcare practitioners may exert their autonomy to practise in a way that reflects their own belief system, whether moral, ethical or religious.

Currently, there are two areas of healthcare where healthcare practitioners may exert a statutory right of conscientious objection. Section 4(1) of the Abortion Act 1967 states, 'no person shall be under any duty, whether by contract or by any statutory or other legal requirement, to participate in any treatment authorised by this Act to which he has a conscientious objection'. This applies to healthcare practitioners working in England, Scotland and Wales. For healthcare practitioners working in Northern Ireland, Part 7 of The Abortion (Northern Ireland) Regulations 2020 has a similar provision.

Where a healthcare practitioner wishes to act upon a conscientious objection provision, they have to prove that they do indeed have a conscientious objection.

It is worth noting that the legal provisions regarding conscientious objection relating to termination of pregnancy do not mean that a healthcare practitioner can refuse to be involved with the care and treatment of a patient undergoing a termination of pregnancy. Both the Act and Regulations have provisions that require a healthcare practitioner to 'participate in treatment which is necessary to save the life, or to prevent grave permanent injury to the physical or mental health, of a pregnant woman' (Abortion Act 1967: Section 4[2]; The Abortion (Northern Ireland) Regulations 2020: Section 12[3]), even if this means participating in a termination of pregnancy.

Additionally, it has been established in common law that the conscientious objection clause may only be invoked in relation to the actual act of the termination of pregnancy. Anything that comes before the actual act or after the pregnancy has ended will fall outside of the conscientious objection clause and a healthcare practitioner will not be able to exclude themselves from these activities (Greater

Glasgow Health Board v Doogan and another [2014], a case which had to decide if two midwives could object to being part of any aspect of abortion, including supervising or supporting staff participating in an abortion). There is also an obligation on a healthcare practitioner to ensure that, where they are unwilling to engage with a termination of pregnancy, they ensure that the patient is referred to someone who will take on the care and treatment of the patient. Until the patient is transferred to the care of that healthcare practitioner, they remain responsible for the patient's care and treatment.

The other area of healthcare practice where a healthcare practitioner may exert a statutory right of conscientious objection is in relation to the activities that are regulated by the Human Fertilisation and Embryology Act 1990, such as embryo research and those related to assisted conception (Human Fertilisation and Embryology Act 1990: Section 38).

There have been attempts over the years to extend the areas for which a healthcare practitioner may exert a statutory right to conscientiously object to participate. The most recent of these was the Conscientious Objection (Medical Activities) Bill [HL] 2017–19, which was first introduced in the House of Lords on 28th June 2017 and progressed through to 23rd March 2018. The Bill was intended to extend a healthcare practitioner's right to conscientious objection to the withdrawal of life-sustaining treatment as well as retaining the two areas previously discussed. It also intended to clarify what participation in the various activities meant.

The Bill did not become law because Parliament ended without the Bill going through all the necessary stages and it has not been introduced in a subsequent session of Parliament. Therefore, at present only the two areas discussed above are ones where a healthcare practitioner may exert a statutory right of conscientious objection.

Who is a parent and who has parental responsibility?

We can think of a parent as being a natural parent or a legal parent. For the purposes of this discussion, a natural parent is one who has a biological or genetic link to the child whereas a legal parent is one who has parental responsibility for a child. It is possible to be both a natural and a legal parent; indeed, this is the case for most parents.

A natural parent is one who has provided genetic material for the creation of the child or, from a legal perspective, someone who has borne and given birth to the child even if they do not have any genetic link to the child, as with some surrogacy arrangements.

Given the increase in assisted means of reproduction in recent years, there is some quite complex law on who should be regarded as the parent of a child. For instance, if a man donates sperm under the requirements of the Human Fertilisation and Embryology Act 2008, he is not considered to be the father of the child. Subject to certain conditions, if a woman conceives through the use of donated sperm, the resultant child will be considered to be both her and her husband's child. There is a legal presumption that a child born to a married couple is the child of both parents.

For most healthcare practitioners, consideration of the natural parent is rarely an issue and it is who has parental responsibility that is of more concern.

Parental responsibility is defined within the Children Act 1989. Section 3(1) of the Children Act 1989 states that parental responsibility 'means all the rights, duties, powers, responsibilities and authority which by law a parent of a child has in relation to the child and his property'. The rights are such things as raising the child according to their own beliefs, having contact with the child, deciding upon the child's name and how they are educated. The duties are such things as providing for the health and welfare of the child and making decisions that are in the best interests of the child, such as consenting to treatment.

In Gillick v West Norfolk and Wisbech Area Health Authority and another [1985] (see **Are children able to consent to their own treatment?** [p. 82]), Lord Fraser made the assertion that parental responsibility did not exist as a principle for the benefit of the parents but rather was a safeguard for the child.

As to who has parental responsibility, by law the natural mother of the child always has parental responsibility, unless this has specifically been removed by an order of a court such as a parental order. Fathers have parental responsibility if they are married to the mother at the time of the child's birth. Female civil partners of the mother will have parental responsibility where the child was conceived by virtue of the provisions of Section 42 of the Human Fertilisation and Embryology Act 2008.

Parental responsibility may also be acquired by fathers who are not married to the child's mother through a 'parental responsibility agreement' with the child's mother; and for children born since 15th April 2002 in Northern Ireland, 1st December 2003 in England and Wales, and 4th May 2006 in Scotland, if the father's name is entered onto the birth certificate of the child. Step-parents can acquire parental responsibility on entering into a marriage or a civil partnership with someone who has parental responsibility with the agreement of the parent with parental responsibility or by a court order. A second female parent is also able to acquire parental responsibility on registering as a parent, through a formal agreement with the mother of the child or via a court order.

Others who may have parental responsibility include legally appointed guardians, those who are caring for a child under a child's residence order and a local authority when a court order or emergency protection order has been made. If a child is in foster care, it may be necessary to check who actually has parental responsibility as it can be the natural parents, the foster parents or the local authority.

Parental responsibility is not affected by the divorce of the child's parents. It is generally removed from the natural parents on the adoption of a child and transferred to the adoptive parents. If a child is placed in care, the parents usually retain parental responsibility, however this is likely to be shared with the local authority under whose care the child has been placed. The Children Act 1989 states that it is not possible to surrender or transfer parental responsibility to another, but it is possible to arrange for part of the responsibility to be met by another. This means that it is possible for someone other than those with parental responsibility to make a decision on a child's behalf with the permission of the individual with parental responsibility, for example a teacher.

Section 5 of the Children Act 1989 states that where someone has care of a child, but does not have parental responsibility, they may 'do what is reasonable in all the circumstances of the case for the purpose of safeguarding or promoting the child's welfare'.

Where someone without parental responsibility is intending to act on behalf of a child, best practice would be for them to discuss this with the person who has parental responsibility, only where this is not possible, such as in an emergency, should they act, or where the matter was a trivial one.

More than one person may have parental responsibility for a child at any one time, as in the case of parents. In such a situation, any of those with parental responsibility may act to meet their responsibility without the agreement of the others, except where this is prohibited by law, as in the non-therapeutic treatment of the child, for instance religious circumcision of a boy.

Where possible, best practice would be to discuss treatment with both parents and to gain both of their agreement to any proposed treatment. Where this is not possible, it is legally permissible to proceed with consent from one person with parental responsibility, except where legally prohibited.

Where a parent exercises their parental responsibility over their child, as in the case of medical treatment, they are required to do so in the best interests of the child, taking into consideration all the factors that are relevant to the welfare of the child in the specific circumstances that are occurring. Therefore, if a healthcare practitioner believes that the parent is not acting in the child's best interests, any decision the parent makes can be challenged through the Courts.

Q Are children allowed to make decisions regarding their reproductive health?

A When considering whether a child can consent to their own treatment (see **Are children able to consent to their own treatment?** [p. 82]), it was noted that children can be divided into two categories: those between 16 and 18 and those under 16. Those who are over 16 but under 18 are able to give consent for their own treatment; this includes all aspects of their healthcare needs, including reproductive health issues.

For children under the age of 16, it was noted that, as a result of the case brought by Mrs Gillick (Gillick v West Norfolk and Wisbech Area Health Authority and another [1985]), if a child is deemed to be competent by a healthcare practitioner (known as being 'Gillick competent' or having 'Gillick competence'), the child may give their own consent to healthcare treatments.

Some healthcare practitioners have questioned whether the principles in the Gillick case should extend to reproductive issues such as contraception and termination of pregnancy because they involve religious, moral and ethical issues that are subject to debate and disagreement. A further examination of the Gillick case will provide clarity on this issue.

The issue at the heart of the Gillick case, and the reason the case was brought by Mrs Gillick, was to determine if it was lawful for a doctor to prescribe contraceptives to a girl under 16 without parental consent where the doctor was unable to persuade the girl to involve her parents in the discussion. Thus, issues related to reproduction were at the very centre of the case.

There were two judgments or decisions in the Gillick case. The first concerns the ability of a child under 16 to make their own treatment decisions when they are deemed to be Gillick competent (this has been discussed when considering **Are children able to consent to their own treatment? (p. 82)** and won't be considered further here). The second refers specifically to the lawfulness of providing contraceptive advice and treatment to a girl under the age of 16.

In making their judgments in the Gillick case, the Law Lords made reference to doctors advising children to abstain from sexual intercourse and, where there was not a reasonable expectation that this would occur, to have the child involve their parents in any decision-making process regarding contraceptive advice or the provision of contraception.

Lord Fraser stated that in his opinion the doctor would:

be justified in proceeding without the parents' consent or even knowledge provided he is satisfied on the following matters:

(1) that the girl (although under 16 years of age) will understand his advice
(2) that he cannot persuade her to inform her parents or to allow him to inform the parents that she is seeking contraceptive advice
(3) that she is very likely to begin or to continue having sexual intercourse with or without contraceptive treatment
(4) that unless she receives contraceptive advice or treatment her physical or mental health or both are likely to suffer
(5) that her best interests require him to give her contraceptive advice, treatment or both without the parental consent (Gillick v West Norfolk and Wisbech Area Health Authority and another [1985]: 413).

These have since become known as the 'Fraser guidelines' and provide the basis upon which contraceptive advice and treatment may be provided to a child under 16.

Initially, Fraser guidelines were limited to advice and treatment related to conception. Over time, the areas which the Fraser guidelines are deemed to cover has expanded to include other areas where a child under 16 may be engaged in sexual intercourse, such as sexually transmitted diseases and abortion.

That the remit of the Fraser guidelines has extended to other areas where a child may be engaged in sexual intercourse was confirmed in the case of R (on the application of Axon) v Secretary of State for Health and another [2006] (see **Do any of the principles of confidentiality change if my patient is under 18? [p. 121]**). In this case, the court held that there is no obligation on a medical practitioner to inform a young person's parents or to ensure that they were informed about proposed advice or treatment in relation to conception, sexually transmitted disease or abortion.

A child under 18, or deemed to be Gillick competent if under 16, is legally entitled to make decisions regarding their reproductive healthcare needs. Best practice, according to the Fraser guidelines, is to try to persuade the child to involve their parents or at least to inform them of the situation they are in, but if the child cannot be persuaded to do so, or to allow the healthcare practitioner to inform them, advice and treatment may proceed based upon the child's consent.

SUMMARY

- Healthcare practitioners may interact with child patients and patients with reproductive issues even though they may not work within these specific areas of healthcare.
- Abortion remains a criminal offence, save for the specific circumstances set out in the Abortion Act 1967 which provide an exemption and a defence.
- The foetus is not recognised as having a separate legal personality until it has an existence independent of its mother.
- A competent woman is legally entitled to make decisions that may adversely affect the foetus.
- The prospective father has no legal rights over the mother's body in respect of the foetus.
- Surrogacy is when a woman carries a baby for another person with the intent of giving the baby to them. It is legal in the United Kingdom but subject to strict regulations.
- A healthcare practitioner who conscientiously objects to termination of pregnancy and/or the activities regulated by the Human Fertilisation and Embryology Act 1990 may exclude themselves from participating in the actual acts involved, provided that it is not an emergency situation.
- Individuals with parental responsibility may make treatment decisions for a child that are in keeping with the child's best interests.
- A child is allowed to make decisions regarding their reproductive health and healthcare needs provided they are competent to do so.

REFERENCES

Abortion Act 1967
Attorney-General's Reference No. 3 of 1994 [1998] AC 245.
Children Act 1989
Congenital Disabilities (Civil Liability) Act 1976.
Conscientious Objection (Medical Activities) Bill [HL] 2017–19.

Cornock, S. (2008) *Conscientious Objection in Medicine*. Unpublished LLM thesis: Cardiff University.

Cornock, M. and Montgomery, H. (2011) 'Children's rights in and out of the womb', *International Journal of Children's Rights*, 19: 3–19.

Gillick v West Norfolk and Wisbech Area Health Authority and another [1985] 3 ALL ER 402.

Greater Glasgow Health Board (Appellant) v Doogan and another (Respondents) (Scotland) [2014] UKSC 68.

Human Fertilisation and Embryology Act 1990.

Human Fertilisation and Embryology Act 2008.

Malicious Shooting or Stabbing Act 1803.

Offences Against the Person Act 1861.

R (on the application of Axon) v Secretary of State for Health and another [2006] EWHC 37 (Admin).

R v Bourne [1939] 1 KB 687.

Re MB [1997] 38 BMLR 175.

Surrogacy Arrangements Act 1985.

The Abortion (Northern Ireland) Regulations 2020 (SI 2020/345).

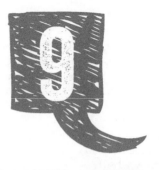

PROTECTING PATIENTS

It may be considered odd to have a chapter dealing with the protection of patients when the protection of their patients should be a priority for healthcare practitioners. This chapter deals with the legal and ethical issues involved in caring and treating patients who may not be able to fully engage with their healthcare needs and thus may be considered to be more vulnerable than the average patient. These patients include those experiencing mental health issues, those at risk of abuse and those whose liberty is restricted because of their healthcare needs, whether adult or child.

QUESTIONS COVERED IN CHAPTER 9

- What is the purpose of mental health legislation?
- Does mental health legislation apply to children?
- How can a patient be detained or compelled to receive treatment under mental health legislation?
- What is an informal patient in terms of mental health legislation?
- As a healthcare practitioner not working in a mental health setting, can I 'hold' a patient under mental health legislation?
- Do the police have a role under mental health legislation?
- What is a place of safety?
- Can a patient be treated without their consent for a medical or surgical condition whilst under a section?
- Do relatives have a role in mental health care and treatment?
- How are patients protected under mental health legislation?
- What is a vulnerable person?
- What protection is there for vulnerable patients in a healthcare setting?
- How should a healthcare practitioner respond if they suspect a patient is being abused or neglected?
- Is it ever appropriate for a healthcare practitioner to restrain or use force on a patient?

Q What is the purpose of mental health legislation?

A Mental health legislation is a catch-all phrase to encompass the various pieces of legislation, both Acts of Parliament and Statutory Instruments, and the associated Codes of Practice that exist in the four countries of the United Kingdom, which make provision for individuals experiencing mental health issues.

There has been legislative provision regarding the treatment of individuals considered to be 'mad' or of 'unsound mind' (terms used in the Acts themselves) for over 300 years. The use of the word 'treatment' should not be taken as meaning that the individual would receive any care or therapy directed at alleviating the mental health symptoms or issues that the individual was experiencing. Rather, it often meant removing the individual from society and placing them in institutions designed for this purpose.

The names of the Acts can sometimes indicate the approach they took to the individuals, such as the Lunatics Act 1842, the Idiots Act 1886, the Mental Deficiency Act 1913, and the Mental Health Act 1959.

The Mental Health Act 1983 is a consolidation Act, which means that it replaced an earlier Act (the Mental Health Act 1959) and amendments that had occurred since that was first passed, and consolidated them into one new Act. The Mental Health Act 1983 applies to England and Wales in full and in part to Northern Ireland and Scotland. Northern Ireland has The Mental Health (Northern Ireland) Order 1986, as amended by The Mental Health (Amendment) (Northern Ireland) Order 2004, as its main mental health legislation, whilst Scotland has the Mental Health (Care and Treatment) (Scotland) Act 2003. All four countries have various other legislation that covers certain aspects of how mental health law operates in their respective countries. Because of the complexity of mental health law, all four countries also have their own codes of practice on the operation of the law.

The Mental Health Act 1983 is the main Act currently in place but was amended and revised by the introduction of the Mental Health Act 2007. Lawyers formally cite the revised Mental Health Act 1983 as the 'Mental Health Act 1983 as amended by the Mental Health Act 2007', though this is quite cumbersome: so, the shorter phrase 'Mental Health Act 1983' is used in this chapter.

Aside from criminal law, mental health law is the only area of law that can result in deprivation of liberty without the consent of the individual. This is because mental health legislation can result in the compulsory detainment of individuals and the compulsory treatment of some of those individuals.

As history in the area of mental health provision in the United Kingdom shows us, this can be open to abuse if not carefully regulated. Thus, the main purpose of mental health legislation is to provide a system of checks and balances on the ways in which the mental health legal system works, protecting individuals from the possible abuses that could occur if it were left unregulated.

Mental health legislation aims to protect the public from individuals who may not be able to control their actions, whilst ensuring that those same individuals receive appropriate care and treatment in a way that protects their rights and freedoms as much as is possible. Protecting the public and protecting patients is a difficult balancing act to achieve and is why mental health legislation is as extensive as it is.

Does mental health legislation apply to children?

Children are specifically mentioned in various parts of mental health legislation. As will be seen in this chapter, children can be subject to compulsory detention in the same way as adult patients.

In the Mental Health Act 1983, there is no lower-age limit at which the provisions within the Act applies. In recognition of this, there are some provisions within the legislation that detail the differences in approach that have to be taken when dealing with a child instead of an adult patient. Some of these differences relate to:

- Case review – a child who is admitted for assessment, treatment, a community treatment order or guardianship must have their case referred to a Mental Health Review Tribunal at least annually; in adults this period is three years.
- Guardianship – a child under 16 may not be placed into guardianship.
- Parental visits – there is a requirement, in some of the provisions, that parents are allowed to visit their children.
- Patient environment – there is an obligation upon hospital managers to ensure that facilities used for children are suitable in relation to the child's age and needs.
- Treatment – some treatments, such as electro-convulsive therapy, are not permitted to be used with children unless the child consents to it.

How can a patient be detained or compelled to receive treatment under mental health legislation?

Article 5 of the Human Rights Act 1998 states, 'everyone has the right to liberty and security of person. No one shall be deprived of his liberty save in the following cases and in accordance with a procedure prescribed by law'. Within Article 5, there are six reasons for lawfully depriving someone of their liberty of which the fifth is 'the lawful detention of persons for the prevention of the spreading of infectious diseases, of persons of unsound mind, alcoholics or drug addicts or vagrants' (Article 5[1][e]).

Mental health legislation provides the legal mechanism for lawfully detaining individuals who are of 'unsound mind'; although the Mental Health Act 1983 uses the term 'mental disorder' and defines this as, 'any disorder or disability of the mind' (Section 1[2]).

There are two main settings where patients may be detained or receive compulsory treatment, these are the hospital and the community settings. All the references to 'sections' that follow are those of the Mental Health Act 1983.

——— **HEALTHCARE PRACTITIONER ROLES IN MENTAL HEALTH** ———

Approved Clinicians are approved by the relevant authorities, for example the Department of Health in England, to undertake certain responsibilities in relation to detained patients; these include:

- doctors
- nurses
- clinical psychologists
- occupational therapists
- social workers.

Approved Mental Health Professionals are approved by a local social services authority to undertake duties in relation to mental health legislation. This used to be the role of the Approved Social Worker. It can now be undertaken by social workers, nurses, occupational therapists or clinical psychologists, but not by doctors.

Responsible Clinicians are Approved Clinicians who have overall responsibility for the patient. This used to be the role of the Responsible Medical Officer. In practice, these are usually doctors, but any Approved Clinician can take on the role.

Section 12 Approved Doctors are approved by the Secretary of State to undertake assessments in relation to the detention and treatment of patients. Section 12 of the Mental Health Act 1983 notes that one of the two doctors making a recommendation has to have 'special experience in the diagnosis or treatment of mental disorder'. A doctor who is an Approved Clinician is automatically a Section 12 Approved Doctor.

HOSPITAL SETTING

Section 2 allows a patient to be admitted to hospital for assessment of a mental disorder where it is in the interests of the patient's health or safety or for the protection of others. An application for assessment can be made by an Approved Mental Health Professional or the patient's nearest relative (see **Do relatives have a role in mental health care and treatment? [p. 195]**) and recommended by two doctors, one of whom has to be a Section 12 Approved Doctor. The detention lasts for 28 days and, following assessment, the patient can be treated with or without their consent for the mental disorder necessitating detention. The period of detention cannot be extended under Section 2 but, if the patient needs to receive further treatment, they can be admitted as an informal patient or under a Section 3 admission.

Section 3 allows a patient to be admitted to hospital for treatment of a mental disorder where it is in the interests of the patient's health or safety or for the protection of others, and where suitable treatment is available. The application for admission is the same as for Section 2 and the period of detention is for up to six months. Section 20 allows for the period to be extended by a further six months initially and then for periods of one year at a time. The patient can be treated with or without their consent for the mental disorder necessitating admission and detention.

Section 4 allows for an application for admission to be made in an emergency. The application can be made by an Approved Mental Health Professional or the patient's nearest relative and only needs the recommendation of one doctor (who does not have to be a Section 12 Approved Doctor). The application has to state why 'it is of urgent necessity for the patient to be admitted and detained' (Mental Health Act 1983: Section 4[2]). The period of admission and detention is for up to 72 hours, which is to allow for a second medical opinion and, if it is deemed necessary, the admission can be converted to a Section 2 admission.

Section 5 is a holding power and allows a patient already in a hospital to be held so that an assessment can be made where it is believed that a patient may be in need of treatment for a mental disorder. The period of detention is for a maximum of six or 72 hours, depending upon who authorised the detention. Doctors or an Approved Clinician, or their nominated deputies, may detain a patient for 72 hours. Nurses 'of the prescribed class' (Mental Health Act 1983: Section 5[4]) may authorise detention for a period of up to six hours ('prescribed class' of nurse is not defined within the Act but is subject to Secretary of State approval, it is generally taken to mean a nurse who is trained in mental health or learning disability). This is to allow time for a doctor to attend to assess the patient. The detention cannot be renewed nor can treatment be given under the provisions in Section 5.

Other sections in relation to detention in hospital relate to transferring the patient to hospital (Section 6), patients being allowed out of hospital on leave (Section 17, see below) and provisions to allow patients who are absent from hospital without authority to be returned to hospital (Section 18). Sections with regard to police powers are discussed when considering **Do the police have a role under mental health legislation? (p. 192).**

COMMUNITY SETTING

Section 7 allows for a patient to be placed under a guardianship order on the recommendation of two doctors following an application by an Approved Mental Health Professional or the patient's nearest relative. As its name suggests, a patient subject to a guardianship order will have a guardian who has authority to make specific requirements of the patient. The effect of a guardianship order is to allow a patient with a mental disorder to be able to reside outside of a hospital but be required to do any or all of the following:

- reside at a stated place
- attend for treatment in relation to their mental disorder
- undertake an occupation, at a stated place
- undertake education or training, at a stated place
- be seen by a suitably qualified healthcare practitioner, or another stated person.

Section 17 allows for patients who are detained in hospital to be allowed a leave of absence. During the period away from hospital, the patient can be recalled back to hospital at any time and may be compelled to receive treatment whilst in the community. Other conditions can be imposed dependent upon the needs of the patient.

Section 17A allows a patient who is detained in hospital for treatment, subject to certain criteria, to be released on certain conditions and subject to being recalled back to hospital at any time, on what is termed a 'Community Treatment Order' (CTO). The conditions relate to the patient continuing to receive treatment and/or any condition that is considered necessary for the patient's health and safety or the safety of others. A CTO is initially made for six months and can be renewed for a further six months, and then yearly.

Q **What is an informal patient in terms of mental health legislation?**

A Informal patients are those patients who have not formally been detained under any of the provisions within the mental health legislation and are admitted for treatment. It is Section 131 of the Mental Health Act 1983 that makes provision for patients to be informally admitted. An informal patient is one who consents to their admission or does not object to their admission. They can include children of any age.

If the child is aged 16–17, they may consent to their admission on their own behalf; if they refuse to be admitted, this cannot be overridden by someone with parental responsibility (see **Who is a parent and who has parental responsibility?** **[p. 180]**). If the child is under 16 or lacks capacity, someone with parental responsibility may consent to their informal admission.

An informal admission has no time limit. The patient is free to leave at any time, however, as with any patient with mental health issues, they can be detained if there are clinical concerns. For instance, under Section 5 of the Mental Health Act 1983 which we have considered in **How can a patient be detained or compelled to receive treatment under mental health legislation? (p. 188).**

The informal admission of a patient for treatment does not mean that treatment may just be given to the patient. The fact that the patient is informally admitted means that, unlike patients formally detained for treatment, they have to give their consent to treatments.

Because a patient may become an informal patient by virtue of not objecting to their admission or lacking the capacity to consent, it is generally considered that such patients should be admitted under a formal detention or via Deprivation of Liberty Safeguards (see **What protection is there for vulnerable patients in a healthcare setting? [p. 198]**) and that informal admission should only be used for those patients who can provide a legally valid consent (see **What criteria must be fulfilled for consent to be legally valid? [p. 68]**) to their admission.

Q **As a healthcare practitioner not working in a mental health setting, can I 'hold' a patient under mental health legislation?**

A In **How can a patient be detained or compelled to receive treatment under mental health legislation? (p. 188)** we identified that a number of individuals have a specified role under the provisions of mental health legislation. If a healthcare practitioner does not fall into one of the classes of individual identified as having a role under mental health legislation, they are not authorised to use the holding powers within the legislation to detain a patient, even if that patient is suffering from a mental disorder.

A doctor may use the provisions in Section 5 of the Mental Health Act 1983 to hold an in-patient in a hospital for up to 72 hours so that they can be assessed to determine if they need to be admitted for further assessment or treatment of a mental disorder. It is important to note that the holding power may only be used to hold a patient in relation to a mental disorder and not for a reason related to a physical illness or condition.

There are strict criteria which have to be followed and the registered medical practitioner has to be the doctor in charge of the patient's treatment. A hospital does not necessarily mean a psychiatric hospital and a general hospital meets the criteria even if the patient has been admitted for a physical condition. An outpatient facility or an emergency department would not meet the criteria as in neither case would the patient be an in-patient; nor can the holding power be used on a day patient as they are not considered to be in-patients under Section 5.

If a Section 5 holding power is utilised in a general hospital setting, best practice would be to have the patient assessed by someone specialising in mental health at the first opportunity that this can be arranged.

Most other healthcare practitioners working in a general hospital would be unlikely to meet the criteria for invoking a holding power under Section 5 of the Mental Health Act 1983.

Q Do the police have a role under mental health legislation?

A The police have defined roles within mental health legislation and specific sections make mention of these. The Policing and Crime Act 2017 amended aspects of the powers that the police can exercise under mental health legislation.

There are two main aspects to the role of the police under mental health legislation. They relate either to individuals who have committed a crime and are suffering from a mental disorder, or to individuals who are experiencing mental health problems but have not committed a crime.

Where an individual who has been charged with criminal offence and ordered to be remanded to hospital either for psychiatric reports or for treatment pending trial and subsequently absconds, the police are empowered to re-detain these individuals and return them to the Courts or the hospital from which they absconded.

Where the individual is not charged with a criminal offence but absents themselves without leave from hospital, and is subject to a mental health section, the police have the power to detain and return them to the hospital.

There are two sections of the Mental Health Act 1983 that require further discussion regarding the role of the police under mental health legislation. These are Sections 135 and 136.

Section 135 of the Mental Health Act 1983 allows for a warrant to be issued, on an application by an Approved Mental Health Professional (see **How can a patient**

be detained or compelled to receive treatment under mental health legislation? [p. 188]), where it is believed that an individual believed to have a mental disorder, 'has been, or is being, ill-treated, neglected or kept otherwise than under proper control, in any place within the jurisdiction of the justice, or being unable to care for himself, is living alone in any such place' (Section 135[1]).

Section 135 provides the police with the power to enter any premises specified in the warrant, using appropriate force if necessary, to search for the individual and, when found, the police are authorised to remove that person to a place of safety. The police executing a warrant under Section 135(1) must be accompanied by an Approved Mental Health Professional and a registered medical practitioner. The individual may be detained for a period of up to 24 hours, unless this is extended on application, so that they can be assessed to determine if they need to be admitted for further assessment or for treatment.

> If a person appears to a constable to be suffering from mental disorder and to be in immediate need of care or control, the constable may, if he thinks it necessary to do so in the interests of that person or for the protection of other persons—
>
> a) remove the person to a place of safety within the meaning of Section 135, or
>
> b) if the person is already at a place of safety within the meaning of that section, keep the person at that place or remove the person to another place of safety. (Mental Health Act 1983: Section 136[1]).

Section 136 therefore allows the police to remove individuals from places where the public have access. Although, where practical, any police officer intending to use their powers under Section 136 is required to consult certain categories of healthcare practitioner, such as a doctor, a nurse, or an Approved Mental Health Professional, to determine whether the use of Section 136 is appropriate.

Once a person is removed under Section 136 and taken to a place of safety, they may be held there for up to 24 hours, unless extended to a maximum of 36 hours, where they are to be examined by a doctor and interviewed by an approved mental health practitioner so that further arrangements may be made for their care and/or treatment.

What is a place of safety?

What is considered to be an appropriate place of safety will depend upon the reason for moving the detained patient to that place. Whether it is for the protection of the individual or for the protection of others will have a bearing on what constitutes a place of safety.

Section 135(6) of the Mental Health Act 1983 defines a place of safety as 'residential accommodation provided by a local social services authority …, a hospital as defined by this Act, a police station, an independent hospital or care home for mentally disordered persons or any other suitable place'.

Any other suitable place includes houses, flats or rooms where the detained person is living, and they agree to it being used as a place of safety and, where others also live there, one of the other occupiers also agrees. Houses/flats may also be used even if the detained person is not living there. In this case, both the patient and at least one of those occupying it must agree to it being used as a place of safety. This includes managed accommodation, such as voluntary sector accommodation, where a 'person who appears to the constable exercising powers under this section to be responsible for the management of the place agrees to its use as a place of safety' (Mental Health Act 1983: Section 135[7][b]).

Section 136A(1) of the Mental Health Act 1983 states, 'a child may not, in the exercise of a power to which this section applies, be removed to, kept at or taken to a place of safety that is a police station'. With regard to the use of police stations as a place of safety for adult detainees, there have been calls for their use to be minimised so that only where it is strictly necessary are individuals detained there. For instance, where the individual being detained is being violent, or posing the threat of violence, to others.

Once someone has been detained at one place of safety, they may be moved to another place of safety if the alternative location is deemed to be more appropriate. For example, the police may take someone to a police station as an immediate place of safety and then move them to an emergency department within a hospital because the person is in need of physical care or treatment that it is not possible to provide within the police station.

Q Can a patient be treated without their consent for a medical or surgical condition whilst under a section?

A A patient who is compulsorily detained under a mental health legislation section is detained so that they can be assessed or treated in relation to a mental disorder. Section 145 of the Mental Health Act 1983 states, 'medical treatment, in relation to mental disorder, shall be construed as a reference to medical treatment the purpose of which is to alleviate, or prevent a worsening of, the disorder or one or more of its symptoms or manifestations'.

This means that treatment which is related to the mental disorder and is anticipated to have a positive effect on that mental disorder can in certain circumstances be compelled upon the patient.

Section 145 of the Mental Health Act 1983 defines medical treatment as including 'nursing, psychological intervention and specialist mental health habilitation, rehabilitation and care'. Therefore, nursing and psychological care and interventions can be compelled upon patients where it is related to the patient's mental disorder.

None of the mental health legislation permits care and/or treatment that is not related to the patient's mental disorder to be imposed upon the patient. This means that, if a patient is detained and needs care and/or treatment that is not related to the mental disorder for which they were detained, this can only be provided to them if they consent or, if they are incapable of consenting, it is considered to be in their best interests. If the patient is a child then consent may be provided by someone with parental responsibility (see **Can a child refuse treatment? [p. 84]**).

Patients who are compulsorily detained under a section may only be treated in relation to the mental disorder which necessitated their detention. In all other aspects of their healthcare needs, they are entitled to the same degree of autonomy as any other patient.

Q Do relatives have a role in mental health care and treatment?

A When discussing the legal basis of next of kin (see **Do next of kin have any legal status?** [p. 90]), it was stated that next of kin have no formal legal basis and are simply someone that the patient may want their healthcare needs and treatment shared with, or be a point of contact between the patient, healthcare practitioners and the patient's family.

Mental health legislation is different in this regard and recognises the role of the relative, and details specific statutory functions that a relative may perform in relation to patients who may be subject to the provisions of mental health legislation.

Both the Mental Health Act 1983 (Section 26) and the Mental Health (Care and Treatment) (Scotland) Act 2003 (Section 254) have provisions regarding the 'nearest relative', and provide details of how the nearest relative can be determined.

The provisions are rather detailed and can be cumbersome to work through to determine whether a particular person should be recognised as a patient's nearest relative, although some general points can be made.

The nearest relative is generally the person highest in the following hierarchy of living relatives:

a) husband or wife or civil partner [or someone who has been living with the patient for a period of not less than six months as the patient's husband, wife or civil partner unless the patient already has a husband, wife or civil partner];

b) son or daughter;

c) father or mother;

d) brother or sister;

e) grandparent;

f) grandchild;

g) uncle or aunt;

h) nephew or niece (Mental Health Act 1983: Section 26[1]).

If there are two in the category, the older generally takes preference. The relative has to be a blood relative so, for example an aunt who was the wife of a blood related uncle would not count. The relative has to be at least 18, unless they are husband, wife, civil partner, mother or father. If the relative is a husband, wife or civil partner, they do not count if they are permanently separated from the patient or have deserted the patient or been deserted by them. The relative has to be living in the United Kingdom, the Channel Islands or the Isle of Man if the patient is living in one of these places.

If none of the relatives above exist or are capable of acting as a nearest relative, Section 26(7) allows for someone with whom the patient normally resides, for a period of not less than five years, to be nominated as the nearest relative.

A patient may object to the person appointed as nearest relative, and the nearest relative can authorise someone else to act in their place. It is also possible to have the nearest relative removed from their role.

The role of the nearest relative is defined in the statutes and this gives them a number of rights and some powers in relation to the patient. These include:

- making an application for the patient's admission for assessment or treatment or a guardianship application
- the right to be informed of any application to admit the patient
- requesting that an Approved Mental Health Professional (see **How can a patient be detained or compelled to receive treatment under mental health legislation? [p. 188]**) review the patient's case with a view to admitting the patient for assessment
- ordering the discharge of the patient, although they must give 72 hours' notice and it can be barred by the Responsible Clinician (see **How can a patient be detained or compelled to receive treatment under mental health legislation? [p. 188]**).
- objecting to the patient's admission for treatment or to a guardianship order
- making an application to a Mental Health Review Tribunal for the patient's discharge where the detention is ordered by a criminal court
- the right to be informed about a patient's detention and any community treatment order, although the patient can object to this
- the right to be informed of the patient's discharge, normally with seven days' notice of the discharge.

The rights and power of the nearest relative are quite extensive and have implications for how the patient interacts with mental health services. The nearest relative acts as a form of statutory safeguard for the patient by both applying for their admission when their condition warrants it and ensuring that any detention remains necessary.

How are patients protected under mental health legislation?

It was stated at the beginning of this chapter that mental health legislation aims to ensure that patients subject to mental health legislation receive the appropriate care and treatment they need in a way that protects their rights and freedoms as far as possible. While the ways in which patients can be compelled to receive treatment have been discussed in the preceding questions, this question examines how patient's rights are protected.

When considering the ways in which a patient can be detained or compelled to receive treatment under mental health legislation in **How can a patient be detained or compelled to receive treatment under mental health legislation?** (p. 188), it was noted that admission to hospital for assessment or treatment was not automatic, is subject to an application being made and needs a positive recommendation on that application.

This is the first of the protection mechanisms that exist in the mental health legislation. Unless in an emergency, an application must be supported by the recommendation of two doctors. The next protection may be considered to be the fact that at least one of the doctors must be a Section 12 Approved Doctor (see **How can a patient be detained or compelled to receive treatment under mental health legislation?** [p. 188]).

Next, the period for which a patient may be detained or compelled to receive treatment under mental health legislation is not indefinite. It is for defined periods and whilst it can be renewed, this is not automatic.

The involvement of the patient's nearest relative is a protective measure as they are someone outside of the healthcare environment who have rights and responsibilities (see **Do relatives have a role in mental health care and treatment?** [p. 195]). These include an oversight of the patient's admission and the right to apply for their release from detention.

The Mental Health Act 1983 refers to the role of 'managers of hospitals' at various points. These give hospital managers various powers and duties in relation to patients who have been detained. This includes a duty to determine the validity of any application for detention and referring the case of individual patients to a tribunal for review of the detention.

Patients and their nearest relative are entitled to make an application to a tribunal for a review of the patient's case. This includes patients on an assessment section as well as a treatment section. The tribunal is able to order the release of the patient if it considers it appropriate to do so.

The Care Quality Commission and its equivalent in the other nations (the Healthcare Inspectorate for Wales, the Healthcare Improvement Scotland, and the Regulation and Quality Improvement Authority in Northern Ireland) is responsible for setting standards and regulating the standards in health and social care provision. Part of the Care Quality Commission's remit is monitoring activities under the Mental Health Act 1983 and ensuring compliance with legislation.

What is a vulnerable person?

Neither the Mental Health Act 1983 nor the Mental Capacity Act 2005 provide a definition of 'vulnerable person' despite the fact that both offer protection to people who might be seen as being vulnerable.

A vulnerable person is someone who is, or may be, unable to adequately look after themselves or their finances or to protect themselves against significant exploitation or harm because of a mental impairment or illness; a developmental, learning or intellectual disability; a physical disability; age; emotional disorder; cognitive disability; or illness or dependency, whether acute or chronic.

The vulnerable person may be a child or an adult. The vulnerability may be a temporary situation, or it may be permanent.

Some vulnerable people may be competent to make some or all decisions regarding their welfare, whilst others may lack competence to do so. Just because someone has competence does not mean that they are not vulnerable. Individuals who lack competence may be more likely to be identified as being vulnerable; however, individuals with competence may still be vulnerable as, due to their physical, mental or emotional disability, they lack the ability to care for themselves and/or to protect themselves from significant exploitation or harm.

Q **What protection is there for vulnerable patients in a healthcare setting?**

A Generally, patients are admitted to hospital for a specific reason and once that reason ceases to exist, for instance because the patient has been treated, the patient leaves hospital and returns to the normal residence.

For some vulnerable patients who may need care because of a mental impairment or illness or a developmental, learning or intellectual disability, this may not be the case.

CASE NOTE 9.1

HL V UK [2004]

HL was a male who suffered from severe autism and was incapable of consenting to medical treatment or making decisions regarding his living arrangements. He had been resident at a hospital for over 30 years and then lived with carers for three years. He attended a day centre on a daily basis. One day he became so agitated at the day centre that he was sedated and taken to an accident and emergency department, where he was assessed and deemed to need admission under the Mental Health Act 1983. However, because he was incompetent and compliant, he was informally admitted instead. His carers were denied contact with him. HL did not try to leave the ward nor was the ward locked. It was asserted that, because he was free to leave, he was not being deprived of his liberty. It was held by the European Court of Human Rights that HL had been deprived of his liberty and that he was not afforded the protection available to him had he been formally admitted under a Mental Health Act 1983 section.

The case and the European Court of Human Rights judgment became known as the 'Bournewood gap' (after the National Health Service [NHS] Trust involved).

This is where incapacitated and compliant patients were admitted to mental health facilities as informal patients rather than under the provisions of the Mental Health Act 1983 with its attendant safeguards. As a consequence, Deprivation of Liberty Safeguards (DoLS) were introduced into the Mental Capacity Act 2005 by the Mental Health Act 2007.

Subsequent cases have confirmed the earlier judgment and added that someone is deprived of their liberty when they are not free to leave and are under constant supervision and control, regardless of whether they comply or not; also, that even if others consider the arrangements to be normal for someone with the patient's condition or illness, they can amount to a deprivation of liberty (P v Cheshire West and Chester Council [2014], a case which concerned whether living arrangements for mentally impaired individuals amounted to a deprivation of liberty).

In Trust A v X and Others [2015] the Court declared that someone with parental responsibility (see **Who is a parent and who has parental responsibility? [p. 180]**) may consent to deprivation of their child's liberty where the child is under 16. In the subsequent case of D (A Child) [2019], the court considered whether this applied if the child was over 16 and held that, where the child has attained their 16th birthday, consent from someone with parental responsibility will not make the deprivation of liberty lawful and permission for any deprivation of liberty must be sought from an appropriate authority.

Where it is necessary to deprive a patient of their liberty outside the provisions of the Mental Health Act 1983, an application has to be made. Schedule A1 of the Mental Capacity Act 2005 sets out the requirements that have to be met in order to lawfully deprive someone of their liberty. These are the DoLS provisions and six requirements need to be met, which are:

- age requirement – the person is over 18
- mental health requirement – the person is suffering from a mental disorder within the meaning in the Mental Health Act 1983
- mental capacity requirement – the person lacks capacity
- best interests requirement – it is in the person's best interests for them to be detained, and the detention is a proportionate response to the likelihood of them suffering harm and the seriousness of that harm
- eligibility requirement – the person is not subject to detention or any other restrictions under the Mental Health Act 1983
- no refusal requirement – the person or their representatives have not already refused the treatment.

Deprivation of liberty cannot be authorised under the DoLS provisions where the patient meets the criteria for detention under Section 2 or 3 of the Mental Health Act 1983.

In order to ensure that the six requirements within DoLS are met, six assessments need to be undertaken. A Section 12 Approved Doctor (see **How can a patient be detained or compelled to receive treatment under mental health legislation? [p. 188]**) can undertake the mental health, mental capacity and eligibility assessments; an Approved Mental Health Professional (see **How can a patient be detained or compelled to receive treatment under mental health legislation? [p. 188]**), or a nurse, occupational therapist or psychologist who is two years post-registration and has undertaken the approved best interests assessment training, can undertake the best interests, age and no refusal assessments, and they may also undertake the mental capacity assessment; and an Approved Mental Health Professional may also undertake the eligibility assessment. The mental health assessor and best interests assessor must be different individuals, and need to discuss their respective assessments.

If the requirements are met and the application is approved, authorisation can be given for deprivation of the patient's liberty for up to a 12-month period, although this should be for the shortest possible period that will meet the patient's needs. No extensions are permitted but subsequent applications can be made, though this needs the six assessments to be repeated. Each subsequent application can authorise deprivation of the patient's liberty for another 12 months.

The authorisation will apply to a particular location and cannot be transferred. Patients may be deprived of their liberty in hospitals or care homes.

It is possible to apply for an urgent authorisation to deprive someone of their liberty until the six assessments can be undertaken. Urgent authorities are made for a period of up to seven days and can be renewed. They can be used where it is necessary to transfer a patient between locations or where there is serious deterioration in a patient's condition that necessitates their admission to hospital.

The protections put in place for a patient who is subject to the DoLS provisions include:

- the use of at least two assessors to determine if the deprivation should be authorised
- that authorisation of deprivation of liberty does not authorise anything else, such as medical treatment
- an appeal against the deprivation of liberty may be made to the Court of Protection
- the deprivation of liberty has to be regularly monitored and reviewed to ensure that it is still necessary
- a supervisory body, such as a local authority, will oversee the patient's deprivation of liberty
- the patient has a representative (this can be a relative or friend) who is there to support and represent the patient, and is able to challenge the deprivation of liberty. They are also allowed to maintain contact with the patient. Where there is no-one who can act as a representative, an Independent Mental Capacity Advocate can be appointed.

It has been announced that DoLS were to be replaced by Liberty Protection Safeguards (LPS) in October 2020. The Mental Capacity (Amendment) Act 2019 contains legislative provisions for this and was passed in May 2019. However, due to the COVID-19 pandemic, their implementation has been postponed and it is anticipated that DoLS will be replaced by LPS by April 2022. One of the areas of change would be that LPS would apply to children aged 16 and over.

 How should a healthcare practitioner respond if they suspect a patient is being abused or neglected?

A Unfortunately, there are many different forms of abuse that someone may be subjected to, including:

- domestic violence
- emotional abuse
- financial abuse
- neglect (including self-neglect)
- organisational abuse
- physical abuse
- psychological abuse
- sexual abuse
- slavery.

It is important to remember that anyone could be subject to abuse, not just those who may be considered vulnerable. Healthcare practitioners may encounter patients who are children or adults, including the elderly, competent or incompetent, who are being subject to one or more forms of abuse, or who may be abusing others.

Healthcare practitioners have a vital role in protecting patients from abuse and/ or neglect. This is because they may have a patient in front of them who is being abused, have access to information that leads them to suspect abuse is occurring, or witness behaviour that leads them to believe someone is being abused.

Abuse can sometimes continue to occur because no action has been taken against the abuser to protect the person being abused. Healthcare practitioners are not expected to stop a patient being abused by themselves, but they can report their concerns. Communication is key to identifying, preventing and stopping abuse. The more healthcare practitioners do not report their concerns, the more likely that the abuse will continue.

When reporting concerns regarding suspected abuse, it is important to remember that patient information is confidential. Similarly, if a patient informs you that they are being abused, this is confidential.

As we saw when considering **How can information be shared without breaching confidentiality? (p. 108)**, if the patient is an adult and competent, it is important to obtain their consent to divulge their confidential information to others. It is not possible to act in the best interests of a competent adult patient who will not consent to you divulging information about them. A competent adult is entitled to make their own decision even if this involves them suffering harm. As a healthcare practitioner, you should advise the patient of the options available to them and try to persuade them of options you consider to be in their best interests in a way that they can understand, but ultimately it is their decision. The only time you should go against a competent patient's wishes are where someone else is at risk of abuse, for example children living with someone being abused, or where it is necessary in the public interest (as we saw in the question **Are there occasions when a healthcare practitioner is obliged to disclose confidential patient information? [p. 111]**).

If the patient is a child or an incompetent adult, you need to act in their best interests. This may involve reporting your concerns even where you cannot obtain consent to do so from the patient.

Where you do report your concerns, you should ensure this is to an appropriate authority/individual. You should only disclose the minimum amount of information that is necessary for the purpose of protecting the patient. You should also inform the patient of what you intend to do beforehand where this is possible.

Every clinical area should have a policy or procedure on how to deal with suspicions of abuse. There should be an individual identified who is a designated safeguarding or child protection lead, or a lead clinician to whom concerns can be reported. You should also approach the relevant person if you are unsure about how to proceed.

If there is any doubt as to whether a specific patient is at risk of abuse, but you have a genuine reasonably held belief that they are, you should raise your concerns with the appropriate individual(s). As long as you are following the appropriate guidance and you only disclose information to relevant individual(s), your actions can be justified even if it turns out that there was no actual abuse occurring.

Q Is it ever appropriate for a healthcare practitioner to restrain or use force on a patient?

A Restraint is defined by Section 5 of the Mental Capacity Act 2005 as the use of, or threat to use, force to make someone do something that they were otherwise refusing to do or where a person's liberty is restricted in some way regardless of whether that person is resisting or not.

Restraint incudes physical restraint such as holding a patient, strapping a patient to a chair or using cot sides to prevent a patient from leaving their bed, limiting the patient's movement, or removing an item such as a walking frame that the patient needs to be able to move around; it can also include chemical restraint such as sedating a patient.

Most people would agree that patients should be able to expect to receive their care and treatment without being restrained or having force used against them. The Human Rights Act 1998 may be said to be supporting this viewpoint. Article 3 provides the right not to suffer inhuman or degrading treatment, whilst Article 5 gives a right to liberty.

Whilst the Human Rights Act 1998 enshrines these rights, they are not absolute and can be deviated from in certain circumstances. An example of this would be where the police need to detain a violent offender; in these circumstances, the use of restraint and placing the offender in custody would be lawful.

There is also a common law doctrine of necessity, which states, 'there is a general power to take such steps as are reasonably necessary and proportionate to protect others from the immediate risk of significant harm. This applies whether or not the patient lacks capacity to make decisions for himself' (Colonel Munjaz v Mersey Care National Health Service Trust and S v Airedale National Health Service Trust [2003]: 544, cases which reviewed the lawfulness of seclusion policies).

Taken together, this means that there are some circumstances where it would be lawful and appropriate for a patient to be restrained or for force to be used. These circumstances are mainly centred around ensuring that the patient receives the care and treatment they need, and preventing harm to others.

Force may be used in compelling patients under various provisions of the Mental Health Act 1983. Section 6 of the Mental Capacity Act 2005 also allows restraint to be used where a patient lacks competence and the healthcare practitioner believes that the restraint is necessary to prevent harm to the patient, and that it is proportionate to the possibility and severity of any harm to the patient.

A patient may also be restrained where there is a risk of someone else being harmed by that patient. From a legal perspective, where a patient may cause harm to others, restraining them to prevent that occurring is seen as being in the patient's best interests.

When restraint is to be used, it has to be because it is in the best interests of the patient to do so and not because it is convenient for the healthcare practitioners. It has to be the least restrictive form of restraint that will achieve the patient's best interests, for the minimum amount of time necessary to achieve its aim, and it should be an exceptional measure and not one that is routinely used.

Any employer or clinical area policy on restraint needs to be followed if a healthcare practitioner is to be seen as following best practice.

SUMMARY

- The purpose of mental health legislation is to protect the public from individuals who may not be able to control their actions, whilst at the same time ensuring that those same individuals receive the appropriate care and treatment they need in a way that protects their rights and freedoms as much as is possible.
- There is no lower-age limit in mental health legislation and children can be subject to its provisions.
- Under mental health legislation, patients can be detained in hospital for assessment or treatment in relation to a mental disorder for their own safety and/or

welfare or the safety of others. They can also be compelled to receive treatment in the community.

- Informal patients are those patients who have not been detained under any of the provisions within the mental health legislation and are admitted for treatment.
- Only healthcare practitioners authorised under mental health legislation can use the provisions in the legislation to detain patients.
- The police have specific powers under mental health legislation, which include removing individuals with a mental disorder to a place of safety where necessary for the individual's best interests or for the protection of others.
- A place of safety includes hospitals, police stations, care homes and hospitals for mentally disordered persons, and the person's own home.
- Patients who are compulsorily detained under a section can only be compelled to accept treatment in relation to their mental disorder.
- The nearest relative is a statutory role and provides the relative with certain rights and powers in relation to the patient.
- Within mental health legislation there are safeguards that aim to protect patients who are subject to its provisions.
- A vulnerable person is someone who is, or may be, unable to adequately look after themselves or their finances or to protect themselves against significant exploitation or harm due to a physical or mental reason.
- Deprivation of Liberty Safeguards (DoLS) exist to protect patients whose liberty may be deprived outside of the provisions in the Mental Health Act 1983.
- A healthcare practitioner should report any concerns they have regarding the abuse or neglect of a patient according to local policy.
- In certain circumstances, a patient may be restrained in their best interests or to prevent harm to others.

REFERENCES

Colonel Munjaz v Mersey Care National Health Service Trust and S v Airedale National Health Service Trust [2003] Lloyds Rep Med 534.
D (A Child) [2019] UKSC 42.
HL v UK 45508/99 [2004] ECHR 471.
Human Rights Act 1998.
Idiots Act 1886.
Lunatics Act 1842.
Mental Capacity Act 2005.
Mental Capacity (Amendment) Act 2019.
Mental Deficiency Act 1913.
Mental Health Act 1959.
Mental Health Act 1983.
Mental Health Act 2007.
Mental Health (Care and Treatment) (Scotland) Act 2003.

P (by his litigation friend the Official Solicitor) (Appellant) v Cheshire West and Chester Council and another (Respondents) and P and Q (by their litigation friend, the Official Solicitor) (Appellants) v Surrey County Council (Respondent) [2014] UKSC 19.

Policing and Crime Act 2017.

The Mental Health (Amendment) (Northern Ireland) Order 2004 (SI 2004/1272).

The Mental Health (Northern Ireland) Order 1986 (SI 1986/595).

Trust A v X and Others [2015] EWHC 922 (Fam).

DEATH AND DYING

Death of a patient is an unfortunate reality of healthcare practice as it is not always possible to preserve life and, at some point, a patient's treatment and care changes from saving their life to making them as comfortable as possible. This chapter discusses issues that arise during care and treatment at the end of life and, when life has ended, that the healthcare practitioner may encounter in their practice. It also explores some of the terminology used in these end-of-life issues.

QUESTIONS COVERED IN CHAPTER 10

- Is there a legal definition of death?
- Can a healthcare practitioner certify that someone has died?
- Who can verify death?
- In what circumstances should a coroner be notified of a patient's death?
- Is suicide legal?
- Can someone lawfully assist another person in their suicide?
- What is euthanasia?
- Is physician assisted suicide different to euthanasia?
- Is euthanasia legal?
- What is death tourism?
- Are Do Not Attempt Resuscitation orders legally valid?
- When is it appropriate to stop treating a patient?
- Does the doctrine of double effect have any bearing on treating a patient at the end of their life?
- How is consent obtained for the use of a patient's organs for transplant?

 Is there a legal definition of death?

 As you can imagine, death is something that is mentioned in legal sources on many occasions and is something that has a legal significance. Yet, despite this, there is no legal definition of death either in statute or common law. It would appear that the law is content to follow medicine and not be tied to a specific definition that may become outdated as medicine advances, or to be involved in decisions that should be clinical in nature.

The legal approach to defining death is to acknowledge that a person is dead when a doctor says they are. This approach was confirmed in the case of Re A [1992].

CASE NOTE 10.1

RE A [1992]

A was a 19-month-old child who was admitted to hospital with suspected non-accidental injuries. On admission, no heartbeat could be detected but he was not deemed to be brainstem dead and he received intensive care assessment and treatment. Unfortunately, A did not respond to treatment and there were no signs of recovery. A few days after admission, A was declared brainstem dead. As a consequence, the hospital wanted to remove ventilation from A. This was a complicated case as there were issues around parental responsibility (see **Who is a parent and who has parental responsibility? [p. 180]**) as A had been placed under an Emergency Protection Order, which gave parental responsibility to the local authority. As we know, this does not necessarily remove it from A's parents and A's parents sought a prohibition order from the court to prevent this. Mr Justice Johnson declared that A was legally dead and it was not unlawful to disconnect A from the ventilator.

The importance of Re A [1992] is that the judge accepted the medical definition of death and that A was dead. This had been accepted in other cases before this (such as R v Malcherek and Steel [1981]), but in those cases the issue of death was a peripheral issue to determining whether an assailant had caused death and Re A [1992] was the first case where a court had to decide the basis of determining death.

In leaving the definition of death to medicine, the law has not absolved itself of any responsibility and requires that relevant processes are followed. This is why certification of death is such an important process as it is this certificate that provides the evidence that a person is dead.

Over the years, many judges have commented in cases before them as to the complexity in outlining the criteria for determining death. In the case of R v Malcherek and Steel [1981] (which concerned the cause of death in two criminal cases), referring to the ability to use bypass machines during heart surgery so that a person may be kept alive when their heart is no longer beating, Lord Lane stated, 'modern techniques have undoubtedly resulted in the blurring of many of the conventional and traditional concepts of death' (R v Malcherek and Steel [1981]: 426–7).

Currently, there are two accepted criteria for determining death. The first is the irreversible cessation of circulatory, respiratory and neurological function; the other is the irreversible cessation of brainstem function, usually known as brainstem death. These are both outlined in a Code of Practice from the Academy of Medical Royal Colleges (2008).

Q Can a healthcare practitioner certify that someone has died?

A Death is a very final aspect of the law, and indeed most other aspects of life, and sets in motion various legal processes such as the transfer of assets from the deceased to other persons named in their will and, as such, is the subject of many legal provisions. Much of this is associated with what happens after the death of a person. Some of it, as we will soon see, is concerned with the actual death of the person and having legal documentation, a certificate, confirming that they are indeed dead and the time of that death. Time of death can be important in the distribution of the deceased's assets.

To comply with the legal necessities and be able to certify that someone has died, the healthcare practitioner needs to be able to issue a certificate that confirms death and the cause of death. However, certification of death is a regulated activity that has its own legal provisions in the Births and Deaths Registration Act 1953. It is Part II of the Act that deals with the registration of death.

Officially, a death certificate is known as a medical certificate of cause of death and allows the person's death to be officially registered, and for a certificate of disposal to be issued. Without the certificate of disposal, the body cannot lawfully be buried or cremated (The Registration of Births, Deaths and Marriages Regulations 1968).

Section 22 of the Births and Deaths Registration Act 1953 deals with certificates of the cause of death and specifically limits their signing to registered medical practitioners, that is doctors. To answer the question: if you are a doctor, yes, you can certify that someone has died; if you are not a doctor, no, you can't.

There are specific rules and regulations about when a doctor is and is not able to sign the medical certificate of cause of death. These change from time to time and include considerations such as whether the death was expected, and whether the death was due to violence or neglect. Where a doctor is unable to sign the certificate, they have to refer the case to the coroner (the role of the coroner is discussed further in the question, **In what circumstances should a coroner be notified of a patient's death?** [p. 209]).

Q Who can verify death?

A In the previous question, we saw that certifying that someone has died is a regulated activity and the responsibility of a registered medical practitioner. However, verifying that death has occurred is not subject to the same legal requirements.

Verification of death means confirming that death has occurred. It has no other legal connotation. The person verifying death has occurred does not need to be able to state the cause of death or the time of death. They simply have to be able to verify that the patient is in fact dead.

There are no legal requirements regarding the verification of death. In fact, legally any competent adult (that is someone competent in determining if death has occurred) may verify that someone has died.

Although anyone competent can verify death, in practice it is usually left to healthcare practitioners to do so. The issue for healthcare practitioners in verifying death is not whether the law allows them to do it, but whether their employer and regulatory body does, and how they can prove they are competent to do so.

In reality, this means that a healthcare practitioner would have to undertake training in determining when death has occurred and be assessed as being competent to determine death. For some healthcare practitioners, this may occur during their pre-registration training whilst for others, it will be an additional role that involves a period of training after their initial registration.

Even if the healthcare practitioner is competent to verify death, they need to check that their employer's policy allows them to undertake the role, and if so, in what circumstances.

Usually, a policy will state the circumstances in which a healthcare practitioner may not verify death. For instance, in patients under 18, those who are not expected to die, where the identity of the patient is unknown, where there is no diagnosis, following an operation, after an incident that resulted in injury such as a fall, or where the death is suspicious. It may also state the circumstances under which verification of death may be undertaken, such as during the night when there is no doctor available. The policy may state the actual process that the healthcare practitioner should follow to determine if death has occurred and, if so, this needs to be followed. Any requirement for specific individuals, such as an on-call doctor, to be notified of the patient's death will also be detailed in the policy.

Once death has been verified, this needs to be recorded in the patient's notes. Again, any employer or local policy will need to be followed, such as the use of specific forms for verification of death.

Provided that a healthcare practitioner has been deemed to be competent in the role and they follow any employer or local policy, they can undertake the verification of death when necessary and appropriate to do so.

In what circumstances should a coroner be notified of a patient's death?

A coroner is a judicial officer who is legally and/or medically trained with responsibility for investigating the cause of death. When undertaking an investigation, Section 5 of the Coroners and Justice Act 2009 states that the purpose:

is to ascertain

(a) who the deceased was;

(b) how, when and where the deceased came by his or her death;

(c) the particulars (if any) required by the 1953 Act to be registered concerning the death.

Coroners also have the power to investigate any treasure or treasure trove that is found.

In **Can a healthcare practitioner certify that someone has died? (p. 208)** we saw that only doctors can sign the medical certificate of cause of death. It was stated that specific rules and regulations exist with regard to the completion of these certificates.

The expectation is that the doctor who attended the patient during their last illness will be the one that completes the medical certificate of cause of death. Normally, this would be the patient's general practitioner (GP) or, if the patient was a hospital in-patient, the consultant in charge of the patient's care or their nominee. However, where a doctor has not seen the patient in the 14 days prior to their death and has not seen the body after death, the coroner has to be notified.

Other times that the coroner has to be notified of a death include:

- Where the death is due to:
  - an accident
  - suicide
  - neglect (including self-neglect)
  - violence
  - industrial disease
  - an unknown cause.
- Deaths occurring:
  - during a surgical operation
  - before recovery from an anaesthetic
  - in or just after release from police or prison custody.

Suspicious or unnatural deaths and those attributable to adverse effects of medical or surgical treatment may also be reported to the coroner.

Additionally, a doctor may seek the advice of a coroner before completing the medical certificate of cause of death as to whether the death should be reported or regarding the cause of death to be entered on the certificate.

The coroner can be notified by the attending doctor or by the Registrar of births and deaths. When notified of a death, the coroner may investigate the cause of death. This can be undertaken through a post-mortem examination or through the holding of an inquest into the person's death. Following any investigation or if it is decided that no further action is necessary, the coroner is able to issue the medical certificate of the cause of death or authorise a doctor to do so.

Q Is suicide legal?

A Suicide is an intentional act; someone has to intend their death and commit an act which results in their death. Therefore, if someone were to take their own life by accident, for instance by unintentionally taking an overdose of a drug, this would not be suicide. Rather, it would be a form of death by accident or misadventure. Equally, if someone attempts to take their own life but fails to do so, this is classed as attempted suicide.

Although it is thought that it was never a criminal offence to commit suicide in Scotland; in England, Northern Ireland and Wales it was a criminal offence, that of self-murder.

It may seem odd to have a criminal offence where to commit the act the person committing it has to be dead, and therefore seemingly unable to be punished. However, there were 'punishments' that could be applied to the dead. These included: the method of disposal of the body, for instance not being allowed to be buried in consecrated grounds and being buried in unorthodox manners such as at night and/or in an unmarked pit; having the body hung in a grotesque manner; the person's possessions being confiscated by the state or church so that they could not be inherited; and the descendents of the person who committed suicide being responsible for a 'fine' in the form of having to pay for any treatment of the corpse by the state, including its disposal.

Where there is a criminal offence, X, there is usually an associated offence of attempted X, in this case attempted suicide. In Christian cultures, those who attempted suicide could be excommunicated. Historically, those found guilty of attempted suicide in England and Wales could be imprisoned.

Section 1 of the Suicide Act 1961 states, 'The rule of law whereby it is a crime for a person to commit suicide is hereby abrogated'. Therefore, with the passing of the Suicide Act 1961, it was no longer a criminal offence to commit or attempt to commit suicide.

In Northern Ireland, it was the Criminal Justice Act (Northern Ireland) 1966 which decriminalised suicide and attempted suicide.

Today, suicide and attempted suicide remains decriminalised and, in the whole of the United Kingdom, it is not a criminal offence to commit suicide or to attempt to commit suicide.

Q Can someone lawfully assist another person in their suicide?

A When the Suicide Act 1961 decriminalised the act of suicide, it established the criminal offence of assisted suicide in England and Wales. As originally enacted, the offence was stated as, 'a person who aids, abets, counsels or procures the suicide of another, or an attempt by another to commit suicide, shall be liable on conviction on indictment to imprisonment for a term not exceeding fourteen years' (Suicide Act 1961: Section 2[1]).

This meant that anyone who provides any form of assistance whatsoever, including giving information, either before or during the act of suicide could be liable for the offence of assisting suicide. A sentence of 14 years reflects the seriousness in which the offence was held. In Northern Ireland, the same provisions of decriminalising suicide and criminalising assisted suicide were enacted by the Criminal Justice (Northern Ireland) Act 1966.

The situation is slightly different in Scotland. As we know, it was not a criminal offence to commit suicide and so this never needed to be decriminalised; therefore, no Act was needed and so the offence of assisting suicide was not introduced. Usually, where there is lack of a statutory provision, we would look to case law to provide guidance as to the legal position on something. As suicide was not a criminal offence in Scotland, there is no case law for us to go to. Whilst there have been calls for the law around assisted suicide to be clarified under Scottish law, this has not been undertaken. The current position is that there is no specific criminal offence of assisted suicide in Scotland, but it is thought that if someone did assist another in their suicide, they could face prosecution under the crimes of reckless endangerment, through culpable homicide to murder.

Thus, across the United Kingdom, there is criminal culpability in assisting someone in their suicide.

Over the years, there have been attempts to have the law on assisting suicide repealed and to have clarification on what 'assistance' means and to reduce the scope of any criminal liability. In an effort to bypass the law in the United Kingdom, some individuals travelled abroad to countries where assisted dying is permitted. Many of these were reported in the national press, as to travel the individuals involved needed assistance in one form or another; there were questions about why those providing assistance were not prosecuted under Section 2 of the Suicide Act 1961 on their return to the United Kingdom.

Additionally, several cases were brought to try to effect a change in the law, such as R (on the application of Pretty) v Director of Public Prosecutions [2001]; however, they did not achieve their aim. A case that did result in clarification of the law on assisted suicide and a change in procedure on how the law was applied, although did not change the actual law, involved Ms Purdy.

CASE NOTE 10.2

R (ON THE APPLICATION OF PURDY) V DIRECTOR OF PUBLIC PROSECUTIONS [2009]

Debbie Purdy suffered with primary progressive multiple sclerosis and sought a declaration from the court that the Director of Public Prosecutions (DPP) had to provide guidance on when he would prosecute for assisted suicide. There is a general code that all Crown Prosecutors use to determine whether to prosecute someone or not, but this had no specific information regarding assisted suicide and so the criteria for prosecution were unclear. The case was heard in the House of Lords and Ms Purdy wanted to know whether her husband would be prosecuted if he assisted her to travel to Switzerland to end her life. The case is similar to the Pretty case but whereas Mrs Pretty did not receive the assurances she wanted, Ms Purdy received the judgment she sought and the DPP was required to publicly identify the circumstances in which someone would be prosecuted for assisting another in their suicide.

The case was heard in July 2009 and, in September 2009, the DPP published the criteria regarding the prosecution of individuals involved in assisted suicide; all cases of assisted suicide would be investigated by the police but the decision to prosecute or not would be based on the criteria in the new policy. It is important to note that the policy does not apply to Scotland as there is no offence of assisted suicide there.

The latest version of the policy is available online (Crown Prosecution Service, 2014). The main factors that would tend against prosecution include the suicide being voluntary, the assistant knowing the victim, the assistant trying to dissuade the victim against suicide, and the assistant acting out of compassion. Factors that favour a prosecution include the victim being under 18, the victim lacking competence to make a decision regarding their own suicide, the assistant pressurising the victim into their suicide, the assistant receiving money for their assistance, the assistant being involved in assisting others in their suicide and the assistant being a healthcare practitioner with the victim in their care. So, a family member who reluctantly assists someone with their suicide is less likely to face prosecution than a healthcare practitioner who assists a patient to commit suicide.

The latest version of the Suicide Act 1961 (amended by the Coroners and Justice Act 2009) states in relation to assisted suicide that:

A person ('D') commits an offence if—

(a) D does an act capable of encouraging or assisting the suicide or attempted suicide of another person, and

(b) D's act was intended to encourage or assist suicide or an attempt at suicide (Section 2[1]).

Additionally, that, 'no proceedings shall be instituted for an offence under this section except by or with the consent of the Director of Public Prosecutions' (Suicide Act 1961: Section 2[4]).

Assisting suicide remains a criminal offence, with a potential sentence of up to 14 years in jail; in some specific circumstances it is tolerated by not being prosecuted, although this is unlikely to be the case for healthcare practitioners wishing to assist their patients in their suicide.

Q What is euthanasia?

A Euthanasia means good or gentle death and comes from the Greek: 'Eu' (meaning good) and 'Thanatos' (meaning death). Something that we would all probably aspire to; I know I do. However, since the 1930s, its use has altered, and it has come to mean the ending of another's life in order to relieve pain and/or suffering. Euthanasia does not suggest killing a patient against their wishes but, rather, doing so at the request of the individual who is in pain or otherwise suffering.

Euthanasia is also sometimes referred to as 'mercy killing', though this sems to be going out of vogue.

There are various forms of euthanasia that appear in both the popular and health-related arenas and press. Some of these terms are contentious and not every-one accepts the differences between the terms being used.

1. **Voluntary euthanasia.** This follows the description above and suggests the end-ing of a life at the request of the patient whose death will be hastened.
2. **Involuntary euthanasia.** This suggests the ending of a life where the wishes of the patient have been ignored or where a competent patient has not been consulted.
3. **Non-voluntary euthanasia.** This relates to ending the life of an incompetent patient; the incompetence could be temporary, such as unconsciousness in an otherwise competent individual, or permanent.
4. **Active euthanasia.** This refers to the ending of a patient's life, at their request, through a direct act. It requires the performance of a deliberate act that causes the death of another, for example injecting potassium chloride into someone else's circulation at their request.
5. **Passive euthanasia.** This is where the ending of another's life is done not through an act but through an omission. For example, through the withholding or withdrawing of treatment such as ventilatory support or medication or the withholding of food and water to patients thereby hastening their death. Some commentators suggest that Do Not Attempt Resuscitation orders may be a form of passive euthanasia.

The terminology around euthanasia is becoming particularly unclear as there is an increasing tendency to form phrases from existing terms, so that voluntary passive euthanasia (see below) is being seen more and more, as is non-voluntary passive euthanasia (for instance withdrawing ventilatory support from an individual who lacks the capacity to consent or not, i.e. is incompetent). However, the use of some of these terms can be misleading as they relate to activities that are not a form of euthanasia but clinical decision making, as we will see in the questions that follow. It is the intent of the healthcare practitioner that is important in these activities.

As an example of a term that can be misunderstood, 'voluntary passive euthana-sia' is used by some authors to refer to assisted suicide. This is a situation where an individual is provided with information about, or the means, such as drugs, to commit suicide. This is incorrect as providing information or means is an act of assistance and is therefore assisted suicide.

Another term that is subject to misuse is 'voluntary active euthanasia'. This is used when an individual is incapable of ending their own life, for instance because they are unable to inject themselves with medication and an assistant injects them at their request. Some authors believe that this is misuse of terminology and prefer to use 'assisted suicide' in this situation.

The difference between suicide, assisted suicide and euthanasia for a competent patient who wishes to die is that, in suicide, the patient needs to do the act, and in assisted suicide, the patient undertakes the act with assistance from someone. The assistance can range from providing the patient with information on how to commit suicide, to providing them with the means for them to commit suicide, such as the provision of lethal drugs. In euthanasia, the act that causes the death of the patient is performed for the patient wishing to die. In assisted suicide, the assistant cannot perform the actual act as this moves from assisting suicide to performing euthanasia. However, in many descriptions of euthanasia, and in some of the terms described above, there is overlap and a blurring of boundaries between assisted suicide and euthanasia.

Is physician assisted suicide different to euthanasia?

As you may expect from the term itself, physician assisted suicide refers to when a doctor, or other healthcare practitioner, is involved in the competent patient's suicide. It is also known by several other terms such as 'doctor assisted suicide' or 'medically assisted suicide' and by its abbreviation, PAS.

In PAS, the person doing the assisting is a doctor and for some this gives the act an air of legitimacy that may be missing if the person assisting is a friend or relative. In general, PAS is seen to mean that the patient's life is ended by administration of a lethal substance, with the doctor's role being prescribing or supplying the drug that the patient will take to end their life, thus facilitating or assisting their suicide. For some, the role of the doctor would be limited to prescribing an appropriate drug in sufficient quantity for the patient to end their own life; others see the doctor's assistance as anything up to the actual act of ending life. If the doctor were to inject a drug, this would effectively be an act of euthanasia.

A key aspect of PAS is that the doctor, in prescribing or supplying the drug, has the knowledge that the patient intends to hasten their own death using the drug and colludes with them in achieving their aim. The doctor has the intention that the patient will achieve their death through the administration of the drug they are supplying or prescribing to the patient.

It is not universally accepted that healthcare practitioners should be involved in euthanasia or assisted suicide and the British Medical Association have opposed physician assisted dying since 2006 (British Medical Association, 2020). It is also currently illegal as it would fall under the law on assisted suicide (see **Can someone lawfully assist another person in their suicide? [p. 211]**) and the fact that it was a doctor, or indeed any other healthcare practitioner, who was assisting the patient would not act as a valid defence to a murder or manslaughter charge.

Q Is euthanasia legal?

A Whatever term is used, whether it is deemed to be voluntary, involuntary, non-voluntary, passive or active, where one person intends to end the life of another, even at that person's request, in the United Kingdom euthanasia is unlawful. Even if the person committing the act is a healthcare practitioner and the person wishing to die is a patient, and the act is being done at the patient's request to ease their suffering; it is still a crime. At the very least, it would be seen as assisted suicide and may even be murder.

The central issue is that of the intent of the person doing the act. What is the person intending to be the consequence of their actions?

When we considered if abortion was legal (see **Is abortion legal? [p. 173]**), we saw that for a crime to be committed there has to be a criminal act, a criminal intent and a lack of a legal defence. If we apply this to euthanasia, we have a person (P) who commits an act that results in the death of another person (D), this would satisfy the criteria for a criminal act. When they commit their act, P intends that D will die as a result, this satisfies the criteria of criminal intent, as causing the death of another is a crime unless there is a legal defence. P could argue in their defence that their act was one of euthanasia and this was a moral act as they were acting for the benefit of D by intentionally taking D's life at D's request because they were in intolerable suffering. However, this would not be a valid legal defence as there is no law that allows P to do this. D can take their own life but cannot receive assistance to do so and neither can P take D's life for them.

It becomes even more obvious when the person who dies is not even involved in the decision making regarding their death. If you look back at the terms used in describing euthanasia (see **What is euthanasia? [p. 214]**) and consider involuntary euthanasia, even if assisted suicide was legal, which we know it isn't, how can it be anything other than murder where one person acts to end the life of another without the involvement of the person who is to die?

As far as the law is concerned, euthanasia is the 'euphemism applied to the (illegal) practice of painlessly bringing about the death of those suffering from incurable diseases' (Curzon, 1994). Although this quotation is from 1994, the legal position has not changed since.

If a healthcare practitioner were to be involved in euthanasia under the present laws of the United Kingdom, as euthanasia is a criminal offence, it would lead to the healthcare practitioner being charged with murder or manslaughter (culpable homicide in Scotland).

Although the above is the legal position in the United Kingdom, there are some countries where euthanasia is lawful. In these countries there is often a different approach to how patients are assisted to die but, in general, they centre around a form of physician assisted death or physician assisted suicide. There are often very specific criteria and regulations about: who can request assistance in their death; how this can be requested; and, how it can be undertaken, including where it must be undertaken, the method of death and who must undertake the actual act.

The current countries where it is lawful to assist patients in their death are:

- Australia but only in the state of Victoria
- Belgium
- Canada
- Colombia
- Luxembourg
- Netherlands
- Switzerland
- United Sates of America: only in the following states
  - California
  - Colorado
  - District of Columbia
  - Hawaii
  - Maine
  - Montana
  - New Jersey
  - Oregon
  - Vermont
  - Washington.

In October 2020, New Zealand voted to legalise euthanasia and this will come into effect within 12 months.

What is death tourism?

There are several terms in use such as 'suicide tourism', 'death tourism', 'euthanasia tourism' and 'assisted suicide tourism'; all of which relate to the practice of travelling from a country where euthanasia or assisted suicide is illegal to one where it is permitted.

In some countries, it is a matter of travelling from one part of the country to another, for instance in the United States of America and Australia, travelling from one state where the practice is unlawful to another state where it is permitted.

Although euthanasia may be lawful in a country, or part of a country, it does not mean that someone who travels to that country, or from one part of the country to another, can automatically avail themselves of the opportunity to have their life ended at a time of their choosing. Some countries have residency requirements that mean a person would have to be a resident of that particular country, or part of the country, for a specific period of time before they are able to avail themselves of the services available to long-term residents.

Depending upon the legal requirements within the country travelled to, the person wishing to die may either be assisted in their suicide or undergo euthanasia.

From a United Kingdom perspective, travelling to another country to die is not unlawful. What may be unlawful is assisting someone to travel to do so as this may fall within the definition of assisted suicide discussed in **Can someone lawfully assist another person in their suicide? (p. 211)**; on return to the United Kingdom, the individual could face prosecution.

Q

Are Do Not Attempt Resuscitation orders legally valid?

A

Do Not Attempt Resuscitation orders (DNARs) are a decision-making mechanism whereby a decision can be made in advance of the need for life-saving treatment, at a time where there is no urgent need for the decision, i.e. the decision can be made before any critical event occurs. They are used where potentially life-saving treatment is considered futile in that it would be ineffective and therefore not in the best interests of the patient.

The use of DNARs, or Do Not Resuscitate orders (DNRs) as they were previously called, has been considered in several legal cases, either as a central issue or peripheral issue when considering some other aspect of care. In these cases, either the DNAR was declared to be lawful or their legal validity has not been called into question and the issue has been one of how they have been or should be used.

With regard to the principles of how DNARs should be used, the case of R (on the application of Tracey) v Cambridge University Hospitals NHS Trust [2014] provides very useful guidance (the comments and quotations that follow come from this case).

The case was concerned with whether a DNAR order (termed a Do Not Attempt Cardio-Pulmonary Resuscitation notice (DNACPR) in the case) had been used appropriately. With regard to the use of DNARs, the court 'recognise[d] that these are difficult issues which require clinicians to make sensitive decisions sometimes in very stressful circumstances. I would add that the court should be very slow to find that such decisions, if conscientiously taken, violate a patient's rights' (R [on the application of Tracey] v Cambridge University Hospitals NHS Trust [2014]: paragraph 54).

The most important principle regarding their use is that the patient is involved in any discussion regarding a DNAR. It was stated, 'DNACPR decisions should be distinguished from other decisions to withhold life-saving treatment because they are taken in advance and therefore they present an opportunity for discussion with patients and their family member' (R [on the application of Tracey] v Cambridge

University Hospitals NHS Trust [2014]: paragraph 42); and more explicitly, that, 'there should be patient involvement in the decision-making process unless this is inappropriate ... that it would cause harm or distress to the patient to be informed and involved in the process' (R [on the application of Tracey] v Cambridge University Hospitals NHS Trust [2014]: 46).

Where it is not possible for the patient to be involved in the decision making, either because of concern that doing so may cause them 'physical or psychological harm' (R [on the application of Tracey] v Cambridge University Hospitals NHS Trust [2014]: 54) or because they lack the competence to do so, their family members should be involved instead.

The decision regarding the use of a DNAR order has to be taken in the patient's best interests. Determining a patient's best interests includes discussing what that patient would want in the particular circumstances, hence the need to involve the patient and/or their family in the decision-making process. The discussion also needs to acknowledge when treatment would be futile.

The patient and/or their representative(s) should be notified of the decision to use a DNAR order and how the decision was reached, including the criteria on which futility was reached. If the patient disagrees with the decision, they are unable to compel a healthcare practitioner to provide treatment that is not clinically indicated because the healthcare practitioner considers it to be futile and not in the patient's best interests. However, the patient or their representative(s) can ask for a second opinion. There is no legal obligation for a healthcare practitioner to arrange a second opinion, but it may provide reassurance to the patient to do so.

The decision-making process and associated discussion has to occur before a DNAR order comes into effect and is placed in the patient's notes. Any DNAR order that is made should be made available to the patient and/or their representative(s) if they request to see it.

There should be a policy regarding the use of DNAR orders available for staff as well as for patients and their representative(s).

DNAR orders can be used with competent adults, incompetent adults and children either in hospital or community settings, provided that the situation in which the patient is in has been considered in the DNAR.

Where a DNAR order exists for a patient, all healthcare practitioners have to follow it. It is an advance declaration of futility and a healthcare practitioner cannot lawfully give treatment to a patient if it is not in the patient's best interests, and futile treatment is never in a patient's best interests.

When is it appropriate to stop treating a patient?

As we know from our discussion of the various aspects of consent, treatment can only be given to a patient when a healthcare practitioner believes that it is appropriate to provide it to that patient *and* when the patient consents to the treatment.

We are also aware that a competent patient may withdraw their consent to a particular treatment or all treatment at any time, without providing a reason. At this point, there is no lawful basis on which treatment can be continued and it must be withdrawn, even if doing so will result in the patient's death. Such requests by patients are not seen as a request for euthanasia or a suicide attempt. As Lord Goff stated:

> there is no question of the patient having committed suicide, nor therefore of the doctor having aided or abetted him in doing so. It is simply that the patient has, as he is entitled to do, declined to consent to treatment which might or would have the effect of prolonging his life, and the doctor has, in accordance with his duty, complied with his patient's wishes (Airedale NHS Trust v Bland [1993]: 866).

This then may be said to be the first point at which stopping or withdrawing treatment is appropriate. In fact, not only appropriate but legally required.

CASE NOTE 10.3

AIREDALE NHS TRUST V BLAND [1993]

Following a severe chest crush injury, AB suffered catastrophic and irreversible damage to the higher functions of his brain and had been in a persistent vegetative state (PVS) for three and a half years. AB was 21 years old and in hospital where he was fed via a nasogastric tube.

> The unanimous opinion of all the doctors who had examined him was that there was no hope whatsoever of recovery or improvement of any kind in his condition and that there was no reasonable possibility of his ever emerging to a cognitive sapient state from his existing persistent vegetative state in which, although he continued to breathe unaided and his digestion continued to function, he could not see, hear, taste, smell or communicate in any way, was incapable of involuntary movement, could not feel pain and had no cognitative function (Airedale NHS Trust v Bland [1993]: 821).

The doctors treating AB concluded 'that it would be appropriate to cease further treatment, which would involve withdrawing the artificial feeding through his nasogastric tube and declining antibiotic treatment if and when infection appeared' (Airedale NHS Trust v Bland [1993]: 821). It was recognised that in doing this AB would die. The doctors treating AB were supported in their view by AB's parents, family and other medical experts. The hospital where AB was being treated sought a declaration from the court that it would be lawful to withdraw treatment from him. The Official Solicitor acting for AB 'contended that the withdrawal of life support was both a breach of the doctor's duty to care for his patient, indefinitely if need be, and a criminal act' (Airedale NHS Trust v Bland [1993]: 822).

Incompetent patients are not able to consent or withdraw their consent if they consented to treatment when competent and subsequently became incompetent. When a patient is not competent to consent to treatment, the treatment can only be given when a healthcare practitioner is of the opinion that it is in the patient's best interests. We considered the concept of best interests when we looked at **How can a healthcare practitioner lawfully treat an incompetent patient? (p. 91).**

Where the healthcare practitioner does not believe that a specific treatment is in a patient's best interests, they are under no legal obligation to provide it to the patient. Many of the cases that provide legal principles regarding the withholding of treatment concern babies or very young children; one such case involved Baby J.

CASE NOTE 10.4

RE J (A MINOR) (WARDSHIP: MEDICAL TREATMENT) [1990]

The court was asked about the lawfulness of withholding ventilation from a five-month-old baby, who had been born prematurely and suffered severe and permanent brain damage. J had twice needed to be ventilated and the weaning process was difficult as J suffered epileptic fits when off the ventilator. Although J was said to have a very low quality of life, he was not actually dying. The medical evidence was that it would not be in J's best interests to re-ventilate him should he suffer another ventilatory crisis. It was held by the court that it was in J's best interests that re-ventilation be withheld in the circumstances of further ventilatory collapse.

The issue for healthcare practitioners, and for the Courts, is in deciding whether the therapeutic aim should be to ease suffering or to prolong life. The Courts have indicated their willingness to accept the opinion of healthcare practitioners when considering the question of appropriateness of treatment, as in the case of Baby J. The Courts have recognised that it is not always in a patient's best interests to be actively treated and that care may be more appropriate.

With regard to the withdrawal of treatment, the Bland case mentioned above is the landmark case in this area. Although subsequent cases have refined and developed the principles established in the case, it was the Bland case where the court first considered end-of-life care in the context of treatment withdrawal and became the legal basis for treatment withdrawal.

There were a number of issues raised by the case that the House of Lords sought to clarify, including: how to decide what treatment a patient should receive when they were unable to consent; what duty of care was owed to AB; and, whether the withdrawal of treatment would be a breach of the health practitioner's duty of care.

As noted above, AB was in a PVS and therefore unable to communicate. He was not able to give, or to withhold, his consent for medical treatment. He had not made any form of advance statement about future treatment decisions. The court was unable to give consent on his behalf, as no-one can consent on behalf of another adult under the law of England and Wales.

As we saw when considering **How can a healthcare practitioner lawfully treat an incompetent patient? (p. 91)**, an incompetent patient may only be treated in their best interests, therefore the court had to decide what was in AB's best interests. The crucial question for Lord Goff was not 'whether it is in the best interests of the patient that he should die. The question is whether it is in the best interests of the patient that his life should be prolonged by the continuance of this form of medical treatment or care' (Airedale NHS Trust v Bland [1993]: 869).

He went on to state that for 'my part I cannot see that medical treatment is appropriate or requisite simply to prolong a patient's life when such treatment has no therapeutic purpose of any kind, as where it is futile because the patient is unconscious and there is no prospect of any improvement in his condition' (Airedale NHS Trust v Bland [1993]: 870).

Lord Keith noted, 'the decision whether or not the continued treatment and care of a PVS patient confers any benefit on him is essentially one for the practitioners in charge of his case' (Airedale NHS Trust v Bland [1993]: 862).

The medical evidence was that treatment was futile in the sense of there being no hope of improvement in AB's condition. It was thus held by the court, 'it would be in the patient's best interests not to prolong his life by continuing ... medical treatment because such continuance was futile and would not confer any benefit on him' (Airedale NHS Trust v Bland [1993]: 822).

Subsequent cases have extended the principles identified in the Bland case so that patients not in PVS may have their treatment withdrawn where it is deemed to not be in their best interests to continue to receive treatment. The outcome of these cases means that it is now considered lawful, and a healthcare practitioner would not breach their duty to the patient, to withdraw treatment from patients if one of the following applies:

- the treatment is futile
- the treatment is overly burdensome on the patient and outweighs any possible benefit to them
- there is no prospect of recovery.

From the above, we can conclude that there are three occasions when it is appropriate to either stop, or not start, treating a patient; these are when:

- a competent patient refuses to consent to the treatment or withdraws their consent to the treatment
- it is not in the patient's best interests to start treatment
- it is not in the patient's best interests to continue with the treatment.

Treatment includes resuscitation, and so resuscitation can be stopped when it becomes obvious that any further attempts would be futile.

There is one further point from Lord Goff that we need to consider regarding withholding and withdrawing treatment from patients. This is, 'the law draws a crucial distinction between cases in which a doctor decides not to provide, or to continue to provide, for his patient treatment or care which could or might prolong his life and those in which he decides … actively to bring about his patient's life to an end' (Airedale NHS Trust v Bland [1993]: 867). The first is the lawful action of a healthcare practitioner caring for their patient, the second is murder and certainly not lawful. As we saw in **Is euthanasia legal? (p. 216)**, it is the intent of the healthcare practitioner that is important.

Q **Does the doctrine of double effect have any bearing on treating a patient at the end of their life?**

A The doctrine of double effect, also referred to as the principle of double effect by some commentators, is a legal principle that has its roots in theology, particularly Roman Catholic teachings.

As we saw in **Is euthanasia legal? (p. 216)**, for someone to be found guilty of murder their intent to cause the death of the person who died has to be proved. It is intention that is at the heart of the doctrine of double effect.

The doctrine of double effect was first put into words in a legal context in the case of R v Bodkin Adams [1957]. This was a case where the doctor was charged with murder, on the basis of alleged overdoses of morphine. In what has come to be known as the doctrine of double effect, Mr Justice Devlin instructed the jury that: 'if the first purpose of medicine, the restoration of health, can no longer be achieved, there is still much for the doctor to do, and he is entitled to do all that is proper and necessary to relieve pain and suffering, even if the measures he takes may incidentally shorten life' (R v Bodkin Adams [1957]: 375).

Recognising that any act may have a good and a bad effect, the doctrine of double effect allows an action to be undertaken to achieve a good consequence even though the possibility of a bad consequence arising is acknowledged.

In practice, the doctrine of double effect means that if a healthcare practitioner believes that a patient needs to receive a particular drug to relieve their pain and/or suffering but recognises that this drug may have unintended consequences such as respiratory depression, and with this knowledge the healthcare practitioner prescribes the drug with the intention of aiding the patient's pain relief and reducing their suffering, they would have a lawful reason for prescribing the drug. If the patient were to die as a result of the effect of the drug, the healthcare practitioner would not be held to have committed murder or manslaughter. This is because the incidental death of the patient, although anticipated, is not the desired outcome.

However, if a healthcare practitioner were to give drugs to a patient with the intention of shortening the life of the patient, this would amount to an act of unlawful killing and would render the practitioner liable to prosecution. This was the situation in R v Cox [1993]. Dr Cox injected his patient with potassium chloride and was found guilty of attempted murder. The defence relied upon the principle of the doctrine of double effect, that Dr Cox's primary intention was to relieve the pain and suffering of his patient. However, the drug used was not a sedative or analgesic and there was no therapeutic purpose in giving potassium chloride to this patient. The prosecution argued that the drug and dosage could only have been used to end the life of the patient. It is for these reasons that the doctrine of double effect was not upheld.

In order to be able to rely upon the doctrine of double effect, the patient must have an illness that is considered to be terminal; the patient must be in pain and/or suffering that requires the administration of an appropriate drug such as an opiate; and the healthcare practitioner in administering the drug must intend that the drug is given to aid the patient's pain relief and/or reduce suffering (the good effect), but the fact that death (the bad effect) may occur is recognised. If the patient dies, this is seen as a side effect of the drug use and not as an intended consequence.

As reaffirmed in a more recent case which concerned whether the law on assisted suicide infringes an individual's human rights, 'a doctor commits no offence when treating a patient in a way which hastens death, if the purpose of the treatment is to relieve pain and suffering (the so-called "double effect")' (R [on the application of Nicklinson and another] v Ministry of Justice [2014]: paragraph 18). Thus, the doctrine of double effect allows healthcare practitioners to prescribe the treatment that they consider correct for their patient, even if the secondary effect is that it may shorten the patient's life. Only healthcare practitioners, who are caring for patients and have a duty of care to them, may rely upon the doctrine of double effect.

Q How is consent obtained for the use of a patient's organs for transplant?

A Since the first kidney transplant performed in 1954, there have been advances in the procedures to retrieve and transplant organs as well as in the techniques used to prevent rejection of the transplanted organ. Alongside this progress have been advances in the type of organ that can be transplanted and now include:

- colon
- cornea
- heart
- kidney
- liver
- lung
- pancreas
- spleen
- stomach.

An issue that has been present since transplantation has increased has been the supply of organs for transplant. The reports from NHS Blood and Transplant, which oversees transplantation, constantly note that the number of individuals waiting for a transplant is in excess of the number of organs that become available.

Throughout the world, various systems have developed for the procurement of organs for transplant purposes to try to meet the demand that exists. Some of these, such as human organ trafficking, are criminal in nature, whilst others such as the payment of individuals for their organs and the use of organs from executed prisoners raise ethical and legal concerns. Some countries, such as Iran, allow for payment to be made to organ donors; others, such as Singapore and Israel, utilise an incentive scheme whereby those who agree to donate their organs after their death hold a priority status on a waiting list if they need to receive a transplant.

In the United Kingdom, it is not possible to 'buy' an organ for the purpose of transplant. Section 32 of the Human Tissue Act 2004 prohibits 'commercial dealings in human material for transplantation'. There are two methods of procuring organs for transplant in the United Kingdom; these being from a live donor or a dead donor.

Live donations are usually of a kidney or part of a liver. Whilst a live donation can be made by someone without specifying who the intended recipient is, it is more usual for the donor to be donating their organ for a specified individual, for instance a family member or friend. Where the donor is not a match for their intended recipient, a process known as 'paired' or 'pooled' donations can be used. This is where a donor (A) gives their organ to a recipient (B), who they are a match for but do not know, on the basis that someone B knows gives their organ to A's relative or friend. The chains involved in pooled donations can be quite long as the donors have to be matched to a suitable recipient, and there has to be a suitable donor for each and every pair (donor and the person they want to receive an organ) in the chain.

In live donations, the person consents to donate their organ. They receive the necessary information regarding the likelihood for success for the recipient as well as the consequences of donating their organ, immediately and for their future health, and the surgery for themselves, in order to be able to give a legally valid consent.

With deceased donors, obviously their permission cannot be obtained after their death and so two main systems have developed: the opt-in and the opt-out systems. The opt-in system requires a competent individual to sign up to a register, or similar, whilst they are alive and indicate that they are willing for their organs, specifying which organs, to be used after their death. Until recently, this was the system used in all four countries of the United Kingdom.

The opt-out system takes the opposite approach and presumes that all competent individuals consent to their organs being used after their death unless they opt-out of the system by indicating their objection. As it relies on the presumption of consent, an opt-out approach to organ donation is also known as the 'presumed consent' donation method or system.

The opt-out system is divided into two approaches, usually known as a 'hard' or 'soft' approach. In the hard approach, unless an individual registers their objection to their organs being used after their death, they can be used regardless of any objection raised after the person's death. A soft opt-out system allows the family members to have a veto over the use of the individual's organs; this is said to take account of those individuals who do object to their organs being used but do not formally register that objection.

This is the other time that was mentioned when we looked at **Do next of kin have any legal status? (p. 90)**, where family may have an involvement in deciding what happens to a person in healthcare. The Human Tissue Act 2004 provides for individuals in a 'qualifying relationship' to give or withhold consent regarding donation of organs. The relationship between an individual and the deceased is ranked in a hierarchy and the person highest in the hierarchy is the one who should be consulted. The hierarchy is stated as:

(a) spouse, civil partner or partner

(b) parent or child

(c) brother or sister

(d) grandparent or grandchild

(e) child of a person falling within (c)

(f) stepfather or stepmother

(g) half-brother or half-sister

(h) friend of longstanding (Human Tissue Act 2004: Section 27[4]).

As the opt-out system only applies to competent adults, those who are either under 18 or who lacked competence for a significant period of time before their death, will be excluded from the system. There is also a requirement that a person has to have lived in a country using an opt-out system for at least 12 months before their death, otherwise they will also be excluded from the system. Permission to use the organs of anyone excluded from the opt-out system will be needed from their family according to the principles just outlined.

With regard to deceased donors in the United Kingdom, the situation is as follows: Wales introduced an opt-out system in December 2015; England moved from an opt-in to an opt-out system in May 2020; and Scotland has passed legislation to move to an opt-out system and is expected to move from an opt-in system in 2021. All three countries will be using a soft opt-out approach. Northern Ireland utilises the opt-in system and has no legislative changes planned.

SUMMARY

- There is no legal definition of death and the law states that a person is dead when a doctor says they are.

- Certifying that someone has died is legally restricted to doctors.
- Any healthcare practitioner competent in determining if death has occurred can verify the death of a patient subject to any employer policy.
- There are specific occasions when the coroner needs to be notified of the death of a patient. This allows the coroner to investigate the cause of death.
- Suicide is when someone intentionally ends their own life. In the United Kingdom, suicide is legal.
- Assisted suicide is illegal in the United Kingdom but, in certain specified circumstances, is tolerated by not being prosecuted. Healthcare practitioners who assist with their patient's suicide are more likely to face prosecution.
- 'Euthanasia' refers to a situation where one person intentionally takes the life of another, at that person's request, usually to relieve intolerable pain and/or suffering.
- Physician assisted suicide is illegal in the United Kingdom and is a form of assisted suicide where the assistance comes from a doctor, or other healthcare practitioner, and is usually taken to mean that the patient's life will be ended by a lethal dose of drug prescribed or supplied by the healthcare practitioner.
- Euthanasia is illegal in the United Kingdom. There are some countries around the world where it is lawful.
- 'Death tourism' refers to someone travelling to another country in order to make use of the lawful mechanisms available there to end their life.
- Do Not Attempt Resuscitation orders are legally valid but require certain criteria to be met before they are put into place, such as discussing their use with the patient.
- Treatment may be withheld or withdrawn from patients where a competent patient will not consent to it; or where it is not considered to be in the patient's best interests for them to receive or continue to receive it.
- Recognising that any act may have a good and a bad effect, the doctrine of double effect is undertaken to achieve the good consequence even though the possibility of the bad consequence arising is acknowledged.
- Organs can be donated from live donors if they consent and from deceased donors either through a system where they register before their death or through a process of presumed consent unless they object to this.

REFERENCES

Academy of Medical Royal Colleges (2008) *A Code of Practice for the Diagnosis and Confirmation of Death*. Academy of Medical Royal Colleges: London.
Airedale NHS Trust v Bland [1993] 1 All ER 821.
Births and Deaths Registration Act 1953
British Medical Association (2020) *The BMA's position on physician-assisted dying*. Available at www.bma.org.uk/advice-and-support/ethics/end-of-life/the-bmas-position-on-physician-assisted-dying
Coroners and Justice Act 2009.

Criminal Justice Act (Northern Ireland) 1966.

Crown Prosecution Service (2014) *Suicide: Policy for Prosecutors in Respect of Cases of Encouraging or Assisting Suicide*: Available at: www.cps.gov.uk/legal-guidance/suicide-policy-prosecutors-respect-cases-encouraging-or-assisting-suicide.

Curzon, L.B. (1994) *Dictionary of Law* (4th edition). Pitman Publishing: London.

Human Tissue Act 2004.

R v Bodkin Adams [1957] Crim LR 365.

R v Cox [1993] 12 BMLR 38.

R v Malcherek and Steel [1981] 2 All ER 422.

Re A [1992] 3 Med LR 303.

Re J (a minor) (wardship: medical treatment) [1990] 3 All ER 930.

R (on the application of Nicklinson and another) v Ministry of Justice [2014] UKSC 38.

R (on the application of Pretty) v Director of Public Prosecutions [2001] UKHL 61.

R (on the application of Purdy) v Director of Public Prosecutions [2009] UKHL 45.

R (on the application of Tracey) v Cambridge University Hospitals NHS Trust [2014] EWCA Civ 822.

Suicide Act 1961.

The Registration of Births, Deaths and Marriages Regulations 1968 (SI 1968/2049).

A FINAL QUESTION

Q Can you summarise this book in one paragraph?

A Of course, I can! I can give you one final thought to take away.

After reading this book, if you have read it all that is, I hope that you will have gathered that the single most important thing that a healthcare practitioner has to consider in relation to their patient is: what is in this patient's best interests at this specific point in time? If you ask yourself this question, you can't go too wrong.

Oh, one other thought; so that's two final thoughts. Be reasonable in everything you do. By which I mean, do what other healthcare practitioners would consider to be reasonable in the circumstances you find yourself. If your actions are considered reasonable by others, you will probably be meeting the required standard.

To answer the question: apparently no, I can't, but I can do it in two, if that is OK.